# Breastfeeding in Hospital

'Breast is best' is today's prevailing mantra. However, women – particularly first-time mothers – frequently feel unsupported when they come to feed their baby. This new experience often takes place in the impersonal and medicalised surroundings of a hospital maternity ward where women are 'seen to' by overworked midwives.

Using a UK-based ethnographic study and interview material this book provides a new, radical and critical perspective on the ways in which women experience breastfeeding in hospitals. It highlights that, in spite of heavy promotion of breastfeeding, there is often a lack of support for women who begin to breastfeed in hospitals, thus challenging the current system of postnatal care within a culture in which neither service user nor service provider feels satisfied.

Incorporating recommendations for policy and practice on infant feeding, *Breastfeeding in Hospital* is highly relevant to health professionals and breastfeeding supporters as well as to students in health and social care, medical anthropology and medical sociology as it explores practice issues while contextualising them within a broad social, political and economic context.

**Dr Fiona Dykes** is Reader in Maternal and Infant Health and leads the Maternal and Infant Nutrition and Nurture Unit (MAINN) at University of Central Lancashire, UK.

# Breastfeeding in Hospital

## Mothers, midwives and the production line

Fiona Dykes

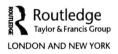
Routledge
Taylor & Francis Group

LONDON AND NEW YORK

First published 2006 by Routledge
2 Park Square, Milton Park, Abingdon, Oxon, OX14 4RN

Simultaneously published in the USA and Canada
by Routledge
270 Madison Ave, New York, NY 10016

Transferred to Digital Printing 2007

*Routledge is an imprint of the Taylor & Francis Group, an informa business*

© 2006 Fiona Dykes

Typeset in Times by
GreenGate Publishing Services, Tonbridge, Kent
Printed and bound in Great Britain by
TJI Digital, Padstow, Cornwall

*British Library Cataloguing in Publication Data*
A catalogue record for this book is available from the British Library

*Library of Congress Cataloging in Publication Data*
Dykes, Fiona.
Breastfeeding in hospital : mothers, midwives, and the production line /
Fiona Dykes.
    p. ; cm.
    Includes bibliographical references and index.
    ISBN 0-415-39575-5 (hardback) – ISBN 0-415-39576-3 (pbk.)
        1. Breastfeeding–Great Britain. I. Title.
[DNLM: 1. Breast Feeding–psychology–England. 2. Breast Feeding–
ethnology–England. 3. Hospital Units–England. 4. Mid-wifery–England.
5. Mothers–psychology–England. WS 125

D996b 2007]
RJ216.D95 2007
649'.33–dc22

                                              2006011915

ISBN10: 0-415-39575-5 (hbk)    ISBN13: 978-0-415-39575-5 (hbk)
ISBN10: 0-415-39576-3 (pbk)    ISBN13: 978-0-415-39576-2 (pbk)
ISBN10: 0-203-96890-5 (ebk)    ISBN13: 978-0-203-96890-1 (ebk)

# Contents

# Foreword

*Mavis Kirkham*

Breastfeeding is not something we, as a society, do well, despite the knowledge that it is 'best'. Department of Health breastfeeding statistics demonstrate this, as do women's stories of their 'failure' to breastfeed or their insufficient milk supply.

In recent years, researchers and midwives have made considerable efforts to increase breastfeeding rates. Women have been provided with information, leaflets abound and experts have ensured that babies are correctly positioned and attached at the breast. Yet breastfeeding rates have changed little and midwives, understaffed and overstretched, sometimes lose heart, as do so many mothers.

This book is important because it helps us to see with fresh eyes, like all good ethnographies of local, rather than exotic, subject areas. It shows what the setting and its culture feel like to those involved: how breastfeeding on the postnatal ward is experienced by new mothers and midwives. The picture conveyed makes me sad, but it feels accurate to me as a midwife and as a mother.

Beyond accurate description and sensitive use of women's words, a key strength of this study is how breastfeeding on the postnatal ward is skilfully placed in its theoretical and historical context. Industrial concepts of time and production are clearly identified and explored.

If we have to understand our world in order to change it, Fiona Dykes has performed a great service to all of us seeking to improve mothers' experience of breastfeeding. Her analysis identifies key conceptual tools which may be used to bring about the radical change that she envisages at the end of the book.

There is a natural tendency, when faced with a problem, to go on doing more of what we normally do. Midwives are constantly urged to do more, which creates frustration and guilt for all concerned and is not conducive to problem solving. This book demonstrates how a very different approach is needed. The analysis develops the growing critique of the culture of maternity services, which is rarely applied to postnatal services. It should be read by policymakers.

An industrial model ill fits the establishment of the essentially nurturing and nourishing relationship which is breastfeeding. NHS structures, cultures and priorities are not good for relationships. Yet, relationships sustain all of us, especially new mothers and babies. In presenting and analysing these contradictions, this book has a relevance way beyond breastfeeding.

Mavis Kirkham, University of Sheffield, 2006

# Preface

## Breastfeeding in hospital: a production line experience?

The promotion of breastfeeding as the optimum infant feeding practice has become a major aspect of the international public health agenda. Breastfeeding is a uniquely female activity that brings women into altered experiences of time, space, relationships and their body. However, within many industrialised communities women commence breastfeeding within a highly medicalised setting, the hospital. This presents a particular set of challenges to breastfeeding women and those endeavouring to support them.

The book describes a critical ethnographic study that focuses upon the experiences of breastfeeding women in hospitals in England and illuminates the experiences of midwives working with breastfeeding women in this medicalised setting. Providing for another's needs in a culture that focuses upon 'racing against the clock' leads to both breastfeeding women and midwives feeling like they are on a production line and experiencing breastfeeding and caring respectively in terms of demand and efficient supply. The book suggests that it is time for: a reconsideration of the way in which we understand and experience our bodies as women; a re-conceptualisation of women's time; a reconfiguration of knowledge about breastfeeding; a re-look at mother–baby and midwife–mother relationships; and finally, a relocation of the place in which women commence their breastfeeding journey.

This research-based book brings a new perspective to the field of infant and young child feeding by illuminating the ways in which breastfeeding has become medicalised and institutionally regulated. The specific focus is upon the hospital setting in a western industrialised country. The book will appeal to researchers and students in anthropology, medical sociology, women's studies, midwifery, medicine and nursing. It will also be of particular interest to voluntary breastfeeding supporters, lactation consultants and women utilising maternity services.

# Acknowledgements

Many people have contributed to the writing of this book and I thank you all. I would like to give special thanks to Professor Mavis Kirkham at the University of Sheffield, for supporting me from my early conceptualisation of this project to final completion. She helped me to cope with the unpredictability and uncertainty of the early stages of ethnographic field work and she challenged me to expand and extend the ways in which I interpreted and presented the data. Many thanks go to the participants in the study, both mothers and midwives, for allowing me to observe, interview and discuss issues with them at a time when they were coping with many other pressures and challenges.

I would like to thank the Dean of the Faculty of Health, Eileen Martin, and the Head of the Department of Midwifery Studies, Margaret Morgan, at the University of Central Lancashire, for providing me with sabbatical time in which I conducted much of the in-depth ethnographic fieldwork. Thanks to those who carried out some of my teaching and related activities while I was on sabbatical to include Victoria Hall Moran, Kate Dinwoodie, Soo Downe, Denis Walsh and Pat Donovan. Special thanks go to my colleagues Kate Dinwoodie, Dawne Gurbutt and Victoria Hall Moran for their friendship, support and encouragement. I thank Dawne, Victoria, Sue Stout and Jane Wright for their helpful comments on the draft version of this book.

I developed some of my thinking for this book during a lecture tour in Australia and New Zealand in 2003. The team I travelled and presented with included Mavis Kirkham, Ruth Deery, Mary Smale, Linda Ball and Angie Sherridan. We presented at: University of Technology, Sydney; the National Association of Childbirth Educator's (NACE) conference in Sydney; the Australian Breastfeeding Association conference in Melbourne; and Massey University, New Zealand. The opportunity to discuss research with our hosts and associates in Australia and New Zealand was tremendous. These people included Lesley Barclay, Virginia Schmied, Cheryl Benn, Barbara Glare, Athena Sheehan, Lin Lock and Sheila Kitzinger who was a keynote speaker at the Sydney and Melbourne conferences.

Aspects of the book appear in shortened versions in two publications: Dykes (2005a) '"Supply" and "Demand": breastfeeding as labour'. *Social Science & Medicine* 60 (10): 2283–2293; and Dykes (2005b) 'A critical ethnographic study of encounters between midwives and breastfeeding women on postnatal wards'. *Midwifery* 21: 241–252. This is permitted within the Elsevier copyright agreement that allows an author to 'prepare other derivative works, to extend the article into book-length form, or to otherwise re-use portions or excerpts in other works, with full acknowledgement of its original publication in the journal'.

Many thanks go to Steve and our three children, Colin, Steffi and Andrea, who have lived the experience of writing this book with me and have supported me in so many ways. I also thank my parents, Sally and Michael, for helping with my children and for providing me with the house that belonged to my grandmother in which to write. Without this quiet and safe haven I do not think I could have completed this work.

# Introduction

## It is about time

Over the past century infant feeding practices within industrialised countries have become increasingly institutionally regulated and notions of how best to feed a baby have become ideologically pervasive. Authoritative knowledge on infant feeding has been constructed, reconstructed and dismantled, sometimes settling for a time, then moving on and shifting. Women's (re)productive experiences have been reconstituted and reconfigured within a profoundly medicalised setting, the hospital. Within this setting infant feeding practices may be regulated, supervised and controlled.

Breastfeeding is a uniquely female embodied activity that brings a woman into altered experiences of temporal and spatial dimensions and new relationships with her baby and others. Breastfeeding is a culturally mediated bio-psychosocial activity and as such has been studied in many academic disciplines ranging from biomedicine, nutrition, midwifery, nursing, politics, sociology, anthropology, psychology and medical geography. There are now several academic journals devoted specifically to the subject and many guide books. Breastfeeding has also become the focus of considerable political activity.

My deliberate use of the word 'breastfeeding' as detached from those who do it reflects the predominant focus of many academics. This centres upon breastfeeding as a health behaviour of considerable importance to maternal and child health. While this is one crucial perspective it is only during the past two decades that researchers have started to ask the question, what is the experience like for *women?* How do they negotiate this experience and what are the constraints upon women from *their* perspectives? While these questions are slowly being understood, the research tends to be discipline-bound. For example, sociologists and feminists exercise caution with regard to the physical aspects of breastfeeding as this may be seen to cross into biological domains and risk a return to essentialism. However, the study of women's experiences of breastfeeding provides exciting and unique opportunities to cross interdisciplinary and theoretical boundaries. With the above considerations in mind, I now highlight my personal journey towards writing this book followed by a brief outline of each chapter.

I was breastfed by my mother, Sally, for three months until she got mastitis and was advised to discontinue. I have little recall of other vicarious experiences related to breastfeeding until I became a student midwife in the south of England. My early reflections on women breastfeeding in a hospital and their encounters with midwives are summed up in a constructed scenario:

> The setting is a ward in a maternity unit in the south of England in the 1980s. Mothers are 'arranged' in two long rows, sitting up 'nicely' in neatly made beds with their quiet babies lying alongside them in perspex cots. The noisy and unruly babies are elsewhere in a nursery. One of the mothers, still sedated and shocked from a traumatic birth, calls for help with her crying baby. The midwife bustles in and purposefully looking up at the large clock, asserts that it is not time for a breastfeed yet and that she will settle the baby in the nursery. The mother looking half bewildered, half-relieved sits back against her neat pillows and watches the postnatal ward 'world' go by. About an hour later the midwife returns; it is now time for a breastfed. The mother rouses herself and sits up in bed for the feed. The midwife, having enquired as to which breast the woman last fed from, grasps her other breast and pushes the baby on to it. The mother, hands by her side, has a strangely detached look in her eyes as if this was neither a part of her nor even happening to her. The baby, having cried for an hour in the nursery, is neither interested nor energetic, and eventually the midwife 'gives up' and deposits the baby unceremoniously back into the cot to sleep off her exhaustion. When the baby wakes again, the midwife again tries to 'fix' her on, and after a further failed attempt, pricks the baby's heel to test her blood sugar level and then announces that the baby needs some milk and that she must give some formula. I watch her collect the ready-made, packaged and labelled bottle, screw on the teat and sit herself in the chair beside the mother. The teat is pushed into the baby's mouth and the baby duly sucks. Each time she stops sucking the midwife 'rattles' the teat in her mouth to keep the baby going. When the procedure is finished the midwife returns the stunned but satiated baby to the cot and announces to the mother that she has taken 30 mls and will be fine. She documents the time and quantity on the chart at the end of the bed, also noting that the baby had passed urine but not meconium. She reorganises the mother's pillows and assists her to reposition herself comfortably and neatly. Order has been restored and mother and baby are looking 'nice', quiet and tidy.

Witnessing scenarios like this started a profound questioning in me as to what had become of the fundamentally female experiences of birth and breastfeeding and what had happened to midwives. What would happen to me if I stayed in this system? A few months after qualifying as a midwife I joined a pioneer team of midwives providing continuity of carer to women. We grew to know the women and they came to trust and relate to us. However, this experience was short-lived as I then moved to the north of England. On commencing work in a northern maternity unit I felt like I had entered a time warp and arrived in the 1960s. I moved into a local housing estate in a socially deprived area for the first few months. The deck access flats have since been condemned and demolished. They were cold, isolated, grey and seriously depressing. In the maternity unit I power-fully re-experienced the frustrations and tensions that had been building up when I was a student midwife. The combination of the aversive living conditions and the hostile maternity environment strengthened both my political convictions and my desire to challenge the current maternity system and the ways in which birth and breastfeeding were 'managed'. This led to a gradual journey into the relative 'safety' of education where I felt, probably somewhat naively, that I could support 'future' midwives in questioning, challenging and changing the system.

In 1990 I gave birth to my son Colin. The experience of breastfeeding Colin was highly challenging for the first three months with episodes of nipple thrush and mastitis punctuating the journey combined with the pressures related to being a new mother. However, after this time I moved onto a profound relational and positive embodied phase during which the experience became increasingly empowering and indeed transformative. Colin stopped breastfeeding at around fourteen months, of his own accord. My second child, Stephanie, was born in 1992 and I breastfed her for sixteen months. My third child, Andrea, was born in 1994 and I breastfed her until she was three-and-a-half years old. I can remember reflecting at various stages during this period in my life upon the experiences of other women, knowing that very few women reached the point at which, in my case, the challenges of breastfeeding were replaced by tremendous fulfilment.

These experiences were key in my developing a particular interest in the global social, political and economic influences upon infant feeding practices. I developed a university module on breastfeeding that I subsequently led and taught (Dykes 1995). This was the first such module to become a compulsory part of undergradu-ate midwifery education in England. In 1996 I conducted a hermeneutic phenomenological study into the breastfeeding experiences of ten women at three points in their journey, commencing six weeks following their birthing (Dykes and Williams 1999; Dykes 2002). Seven of the ten women felt that they 'fell by the way-side', explaining their sense of isolation and lack of support, nurture and replenishment. Three women described a powerful and enjoyable experience.

Through this study I increasingly realised that during my own experiences of breastfeeding I had received an enormous amount of social support from my fam-ily and friends and that this was not the norm for many women. As women spoke with me they often reflected back on their experiences of inadequate midwifery support both in hospital and at home. I wished I had started the study from the postnatal ward experience onwards, rather than from six weeks after the birth. Second, I realised the need not only to hear about the hospital experience but to see it. I wanted to understand what is was like for women breastfeeding in UK hospitals at the turn of the twenty-first century, and how the postnatal ward cul-ture and midwifery practices and interactions influenced these experiences. I was also interested in exploring midwives' ways of working with and supporting breastfeeding women. This led me to conduct the ethnographic study described in this book. I now present an outline of each chapter.

In Chapter 1, I focus upon the parallel yet synergistic development, in the west, of industrialisation, mechanisation, factories and biomedicine and how these influenced women's reproductive experiences. I refer to key moments of historical significance through a 'critical' lens, with the notions of ideology and power being located centrally. In line with this critical approach I avoid presenting a detailed and linear chronology, but rather highlight key social, political and economic events of relevance to this book. I commence with the Enlightenment as this era marked the way for a profound reconfiguration of the ways in which reproductive activities were conceptualised and experienced by women. I then focus upon the development and rise of the techno-medical model of medicine and its central arena, the hospital. I highlight powerful and hegemonic influences upon women's reproductive experiences and the way in which the hospital, based on the factory, became the place and space within which women gave birth. I also discuss some of the ways in which women engaged with and indeed contributed towards a reconfiguring of birth by relating them to the complex socio-cultural context of women's lives.

In Chapter 2, I discuss critical moments of significance that have influenced infant feeding and more specifically breastfeeding policy and practice in industrialised countries across the world. This includes discussion around the medicalisation of infant feeding and the marketing of breast milk substitutes. I highlight the hospital as the place in which breastfeeding became institutionally regulated and notions of how to feed infants became ideologically pervasive. I also focus upon breastfeeding within the fabric of women's lives, acknowledging that there are multiple and complex influences upon their infant feeding decisions and experiences.

In Chapter 3, I discuss my critical theoretical perspective underpinning the ethnographic study described in this book. I then discuss the conduct of the ethnography and describe the hospital culture within which women commence their breastfeeding journey. I illustrate the hospital culture with some of my ethnographic observations and narratives of breastfeeding women and midwives. This provides the context for the ensuing chapters in that I emphasise not only the medical nature of the experience for women but the 'factory-like' working conditions for midwives.

In Chapter 4, I draw upon notions of labouring bodies to theorise women's perceptions of their role as breast-milk producers and deliverers and the demanding nature of this role. I utilise the industrial metaphor 'supplying' to illustrate the ways in which women conceptualised and negotiated this role with all of its inherent uncertainties. I then discuss the ways in which women experienced breastfeeding as physically and emotionally 'demanding' in terms of their temporal and bodily boundaries. I highlight the ways in which women, with their central preoccupation with supplying and demanding, sought ways in which to cope with and control for the unpredictability of their bodily experiences of breastfeeding and activities of their babies.

In Chapter 5, I focus upon the working conditions for hospital midwives with the metaphor of the factory, with its notions of production, demand and efficient supply against linear time being central to their experiences. I highlight midwives as the main group of people with whom women engage while in hospital and illustrate ways in which they negotiate and indeed 'process' their work, given the enormous constraints upon them. The impact of midwives' ways of working in hospital upon the experiences of women is illustrated. Case studies generated through interviews with midwives and breastfeeding women and observations of encounters between the two groups are utilised throughout the chapter.

In Chapter 6, I illustrate the striking parallels between breastfeeding women and midwives and assert that both are engaged in 'productive' activities under considerable emotional pressure in a highly public place, open to many observers. 'Supplying' for another's needs in a culture that focuses upon 'racing against the clock' leads to both mothers and midwives constructing ways of coping and controlling their situation. Given this scenario, I discuss implications for practice and policy. I make recommendations for a reconsideration of the way in which women's bodies are understood and experienced, a re-conceptualisation of women's time, reconfiguration of knowledge about breastfeeding, re-visioning of the mother–baby and midwife–mother relationships and relocation of the place and space in which mothers commence their breastfeeding journey.

# Chapter 1

# The birthing of the production line

## Introduction

In this chapter I focus upon the parallel yet synergistic development, in the west, of industrialisation, mechanisation, factories and biomedicine and how this influenced women's reproductive experiences. I refer to key moments of historical significance through a 'critical' lens, with the notions of ideology and power being located centrally. In line with this critical approach I avoid presenting a detailed and linear chronology, but rather highlight key social, political and economic events of relevance to this book. I commence with the Enlightenment, as this era marked the way for a profound reconfiguration of the ways in which reproductive activities were conceptualised and experienced by women. I then focus upon the development and rise of the techno-medical model of medicine and its central arena, the hospital. I highlight powerful and hegemonic influences upon women's reproductive experiences and the way in which the hospital, based on the factory, became the place and space within which women gave birth. I also discuss some of the ways in which women engaged with and indeed contributed towards a reconfiguring of birth by relating them to the complex socio-cultural context of women's lives.

## The Enlightenment

The era referred to as the Enlightenment represents a major turning point in human history: a 'self-proclaimed Age of Reason' that began in England in the seventeenth century and subsequently spread to western Europe during the eighteenth century (Crotty 1998: 18). This period was characterised by the development of rationalistic science as a supreme source of authoritative knowledge. Authoritative knowledge is described as the legitimisation of one form of 'knowing' over other ways of knowing; subordinating, devaluing, delegitimising and often dismissing them (Jordan 1997: 56). The Enlightenment was also the era during which there was an exponential growth in the human population and increasing industrialisation (Pelling *et al.* 1995).

## Populations and production

The Industrial Revolution was well underway from the late eighteenth to mid nineteenth centuries and, as Doyal and Pennell (1979) highlight, this contributed to the mass movement of people into cities. The development and growth of the capitalist economy took place concurrently with its emphasis upon productivity for profit and monitoring of efficiency and outputs (Doyal and Pennell 1979; Foucault 1977, 1981). Indeed, the growth of the population and growth of capitalism could be seen as symbiotic, as argued by Foucault:

> The two processes – the accumulation of men and the accumulation of capital – cannot be separated; it would not have been possible to solve the problem of the accumulation of men without the growth of an apparatus of production capable of sustaining them and using them; conversely, the techniques that made the cumulative multiplicity of men useful accelerated the accumulation of capital.
>
> (Foucault 1977: 221)

Thus capitalism was made possible by the 'controlled insertion of bodies into the machinery of production and the adjustment of the phenomena of population to economic processes' (Foucault 1977: 141). As Fairclough (1992) states, 'modern societies are characterised by a tendency towards increasing control over more and more parts of peoples' lives' with technologisation playing an increasing role (215). Foucault (1977, 1980, 1981) argues that this expanding population and the need for controlled production contributed to the formation of the major systems that he calls 'disciplines', i.e. the military, prisons, factories, hospitals and schools. As the apparatus of production grew and became increasingly complex the growing costs required acceleration in profitability. In this context the disciplines functioned as 'techniques for making useful individuals' (Foucault 1977: 211); for example the individual capable of mechanical work in a factory.

## Rationalistic science as the supreme source of authoritative knowledge

The Enlightenment was the era during which rationalistic science reached a supreme authoritative status, bringing with it an epistemology of objectivism. The essence of objectivism centres upon the 'view that things exist as meaningful entities independently of consciousness and experience, that they have truth and meaning residing in them as objects' (Crotty 1998: 5). Objectivism is underpinned by reductionism and dualism with the former referring to the philosophic view that complex phenomena are nothing more than the sum of their parts (Engel 1977; Marston and Forster 1999). Dualism relates to the view that the mind is a separate entity from the body thus paving the way for the objectification of the latter (Engel 1977; Davis-Floyd 1994). The notion of dualism may extend to a distinction between the mind and objects within the material universe, thus enabling the study of the universe as separate from any consideration of the human mind (Crotty 1998). The objectivist epistemology so characteristic of the Enlightenment period led to the viewing of the world through a positivistic lens so that it could be explained, described, codified and quantified in order to reveal its absolute laws and principles (Doyal and Pennell 1979; Marston and Forster 1999; Crotty 1998). Therefore, during the Enlightenment, reason increasingly superseded revelation, rationalism suppressed and opposed the metaphysical, and certainty replaced mystery and complexity.

### Separating spheres – constructing dualisms

It is crucial to view the impact of Enlightenment thought upon the ways in which women were conceptualised, for as Shildrick (1997) asserts, 'In directing its attention to mastery of the natural world and given the close identification of the female with nature, the scientific project of the Enlightenment may be conceptualised as inherently hostile to women' (26). While, as Shildrick (1997) argues, it is simplistic to entirely attribute separation of male and female domains to 'Enlightenment' thought, the hierarchical separation of the roles of 'male equals culture' and 'female equals nature' developed very clearly during this era. Martin (1987) refers to this doctrine of two spheres by first connecting the development of industrialised and capitalist societies with displacement of production from the home to the factory. This contributed to the construction of public and private domains. The public world of paid work, that is work involved in the production process, came to be seen as separate from the private world centred in the home. Previously, work had been located in and around the home with the extended family being seen as united in an endeavour to make provision for their own needs.

During the Enlightenment, the private world became increasingly associated with the 'natural', that is bodily functions, sexuality, intimate relationships, morality, kinship and expression of emotions. Women, who were seen as 'natural', increasingly came to be seen as located within the private world of the home, as wives and mothers. Their role was one of reproduction rather than production in the industrial and economic sense. The public world, on the other hand, was seen as related to the impersonal process of efficient, goal-orientated competitive production. It was not only seen as breaking away from nature, but indeed dominating and controlling it. This was the world of the wage-earning male who came to be seen as cultural, in contrast and in superior position to the feminine and natural (Martin 1987). Women from poor families were the exception to this public–private divide in that they were forced into the ambiguous position of juggling paid employment and home responsibilities (Doyal and Pennell 1979).

## Surveillance

The development during the eighteenth and nineteenth centuries of mechanisms and means for surveillance of the growing, mobile population described by Foucault (1977, 1980) is particularly relevant. He argues that 'this moment in time corresponds to the formation of, gradual in some respects and rapid in others, a new mode of exercise of power' (1980: 38), leading to the development of a 'disciplinary society' (1977: 209). He argues that 'discipline fixes; it arrests or regulates movements; it clears up confusion; it dissipates compact groupings of individuals wandering about the country in unpredictable ways; it establishes calculated distributions' (Foucault 1977: 219).

To understand Foucault's notion of the disciplinary society it is useful to commence with his focus upon the prison and Panopticism. Panopticism was a 'technological invention in the order of power, comparable to the steam engine in the order of production' (Foucault 1980: 71). Foucault (1977) describes the transformation during the eighteenth and nineteenth centuries from the body as focus for punishment whose severity varied with the crime, to the body being subjected to the power of imprisonment with its removal of freedom. He describes in detail a building, the Panopticon, designed by Bentham, that was circular with a central tower. The prisoners' cells were positioned radially around the edge of the building. The central tower had a window and lighting system that allowed a supervisor to watch every prisoner in the building. Each prisoner was separated from his neighbours by a wall so visibility was one-way, supervisor to prisoner. It was never lateral, thus negating disruption or communication between prisoners. The major function of the Panopticon is described:

> To induce in the inmate a state of conscious and permanent visibility that assures the automatic functioning of power [...]. Bentham laid down the principle that power should be visible and unverifiable. Visible: the inmate will constantly have before his eyes the tall outline of the central tower from which he is spied upon. Unverifiable: the inmate must never know whether he is being looked at at any moment; but he must be sure that he may always be so.
>
> (Foucault 1977: 201)

This means of exerting power created 'dissymmetry' between observer and observed, 'disequilibrium' and 'difference' (Foucault 1977: 203). As Kendall and Wickham (1999) describe, for Foucault, the prison as a form of visibility assisted in constructing the concept of criminality, whilst statements related to criminality produced forms of visibility that reinforced prison. Foucault (1977, 1980) asserts that the architectural design of the Panopticon was utilised to insert this form of surveillance into other 'formidable disciplinary regimes' (1980: 58); for example factories, schools, hospitals and army barracks. These institutions with their large populations developed specific hierarchies, spatial arrangements and surveillance systems centred around the requirement to supervise activities. Thus the exercise of power through 'the gaze' was facilitated:

> The perfect disciplinary apparatus would make it possible for a single gaze to see everything constantly. A central point would be both source of light illuminating everything, and a locus of convergence for everything that must be known: a perfect eye that nothing would escape and a centre towards which all gazes would be turned.
>
> (Foucault 1977: 173)

Taking the factories that emerged at the end of the eighteenth century as an example, we see that individuals had to be strategically placed and monitored, in relation to the spatial arrangements and operational requirements of production machinery, to ensure maximum efficiency and output:

> A central aisle allowed the supervisor to walk up and carry out a supervision that was both general and individual: to observe the worker's presence and application, and the quality of his work; to compare workers with one another, to classify them according to skill and speed; to follow the successive stages of the production process.
>
> (Foucault 1977: 145)

Again, this factory surveillance links with its economic functions, maintaining the link between populations and production:

> As the machinery of production became larger and more complex, as the number of workers and the division of labour increased, supervision became ever more necessary and more difficult [....]. What was now needed was an intense, continuous supervision; it ran right through the labour process; it did not bear – or not only – on production (the nature and quantity of raw materials, the type of instruments used, the dimensions and quality of the products); it also took into account the activity of the men, their skill, the way they set about their tasks, their promptness, their zeal, their behaviours [....]. Surveillance thus becomes a decisive economic operator both as an internal part of the production machinery and as a specific mechanism in the disciplinary power.
>
> (Foucault 1977: 174)

Foucault (1977: 170) refers to 'hierarchical observation'; the extension of surveillance within the disciplines to those supervising:

> The Panopticon may even provide an apparatus for supervising its own mechanisms. In this central tower, the director may spy on all the employees that he has under his orders: nurses, doctors, foremen, teachers, warders; he will

be able to judge them continuously, alter their behaviour, impose upon them the methods he thinks best; and it will even be possible to observe the director himself. An inspector arriving unexpectedly at the centre of the Panopticon will be able to judge at a glance, without anything being concealed from him, how the entire establishment is functioning.

(Foucault 1977: 204)

The connections between the prison, the factory and the hospital become immediately striking, hence setting the scene here. I return to the hospital, as a site for the implementation of surveillance mechanisms, later in this chapter.

### Construction of a clockwork culture

As capitalism, mechanisation and the requirement for controlled production methods developed, the need for precise timing, measurement and consistency grew (Gray 1993; Palmer 1993). The construction of the mechanical clock provided the perfect tool to connect the imperatives of industrial productivity, mathematical measurement and the monitoring and surveillance of groups of people. The desire to control time, and indeed the concomitant control that clock time has over people, is central to this thesis and I therefore introduce a brief history of the mechanical clock.

Cipolla (1967) traces the development of the mechanical clock within the socio-historical context of the economic and technological processes by which Europe gained power in the world. He links the clock's growing super-valuation with the growth of industrialisation and related technical machinery and with the philosophy of empiricism and utilitarianism which 'infected' all branches of human knowledge (33). The desire for power in Europe that manifested in the combination of wars, industrialisation (later capitalism), and the growth of empirical science paved the way for a central and growing place for the mechanical clock. Cipolla notes that many of the early clock-makers were also gun-founders and he asserts that this connection has major significance. 'The simultaneous appearance of the gun and the mechanical clock was both a testimony to the character of European development and a forecast of things to come' (40).

Cipolla argues that it was during the seventeenth century, when the scientific revolution 'exploded', that scientists saw the clock as 'the machine *par excellence*' (57). Their growing interest in the clock led to its rapid technological sophistication. This was also the era when growing numbers of relatively wealthy urban dwellers – for example merchants, lawyers and doctors – could afford watches and clocks which were being made at increasingly low costs. So demand fuelled supply and vice versa. The clock fulfilled the growing human desire to measure time and rapidly became a status symbol. As Cipolla states, people increasingly timed activities they would never have thought of timing. People became obsessed with punctuality and timing, which was seen to be virtuous. Clocks were changing ways of thinking as they replaced the variable times associated with the seasons with a measured time that overrode the former. Cipolla refers to these clocks as machines which like other new machines create new needs and therefore 'breed' newer machines (105). Each new tool then influences us deeply while we are using it. 'The fascination exerted by the machine induces a rapidly growing number of people into a tragic fetishism of the machine' (Cipolla 1967: 106–107).

In the forward to Cipolla's text, Ollard (1967) summarises the tyrannical connections between the clock and power:

> Clocks are the prototypes for all precision instruments: and once they are valued as such and not simply admired as the most delicate and enchanting of mechanical toys the age of industrial innocence is over [...]. If wrist watches and guided missiles are not obtainable at one and the same shop they still to the reflective eye disclose a recognisable cousinhood.
>
> (Ollard 1967: ii)

As Thomas (1992) states, 'Any understanding of time must identify which time and whose time is involved' (65). What evolved during the Industrial Revolution was the notion of mechanical clock or linear time. This may be contrasted with cyclical or rhythmic time. Linear time is commonly referred to as having overridden or obliterated cyclical/rhythmic time (Cipolla 1967; Kahn 1989; Adam 1992; Bellaby 1992; Helman 1992; Starkey 1992). Kahn (1989) makes the distinction between the two times particularly clear. She compares the concept of 'linear time', also referred to as 'clock time', 'historical time' or 'industrial time', with the concept of 'cyclical time', also referred to as 'organic time' or 'agricultural time'. She states:

> The kind of time we are most familiar with is historical or clock time, a life sequence which moves relentlessly forward. In the West we have lived in this kind of time for so long it seems almost impossible for things to be otherwise.
>
> (Kahn 1989: 20)

Linear time, Kahn (1989) argues, is 'pitched towards the future' (21) and is centred around the notion of production which in the factory not only overrides closeness to natural body rhythms and flows, but with shift work even erases day and night distinctions. It consequently exerts control over nature. In contrast, cyclical time relates to the 'organic cycle of life' in which one is 'living within the cycle of one's own body'. It is a time that is 'cyclical like the seasons, or the gyre-like motion of the generations' (21).

The sense of the clock having deeply penetrated society is emphasised by Simonds (2002), who refers to the perpetuating nature of the western dependence upon clock time, as the clock and technological 'progress' have become mutually dependent: 'A cultural ethos (capitalist, technocratic, bureaucratic, and psychologically individualistic) makes time keeping relevant and, the more it develops such foci, the more it creates technology to assess, to measure, to control' (569).

Linear time was fundamentally favoured and imposed by those in power; for example the wealthy upon the less powerful in factories (Kahn 1989; Bellaby 1992; Starkey 1992). It also disadvantaged women in that, as Forman and Sowton (1989) observe, male-centred western epistemologies around time have reached into the lives of women. However, linear time has not simply been imposed upon women, for they have increasingly embraced this form of time within the fabric of their lives. The ways in which linear time weaves in and out of women's lives will continue to constitute a central theme throughout this book.

## Ideological ascendency of techno-medicine

The dramatic transformation of the practice of home-based medicine to techno-medicine in western Europe during the Enlightenment is widely reported (Doyal and Pennell 1979; Lupton 1994; Illich 1995). From the Middle Ages to the late eighteenth century, medicine had been practised in the home, with the doctor attending patrons, as requested by the latter or their family members. Only the wealthy could afford this service and patrons decided which doctor they would select. As it was the patrons who summoned doctors, they retained an autonomous and dominant position within the relationship. The fundamental belief system regarding health that persisted during this era could be summarised as 'vitalism', a belief in the wholeness and unity of the human person (Doyal and Pennell 1979: 33). The era of home-based medicine and holism came to an end through two key and interconnected changes, the scientification of medicine and the establishment of the hospital, which I discuss in turn. Before doing this, I clarify my perspective on techno-medicine.

I assert that techno-medicine is hegemonically connected with industrialisation (Doyal and Pennell 1979, Illich 1995), the super-valuation of technology (Doyal and Pennell 1979; Davis-Floyd 1992, 1994) and capitalism (Doyal and Pennell 1979; Davis-Floyd 1992, 1994). I agree with Doyal and Pennell (1979) who describe the western health system as functioning as a powerful agency of 'socialisation and social control' (42). By claiming a scientific basis for its practice, techno-medicine is part of the machinery by which capitalism is legitimated, in that capitalism is also aligned ideologically to scientific and technologic progress. Like mature capitalism, the health system involves relationships that are 'bureaucratic, hierarchical and authoritarian' (Doyal and Pennell 1979: 43). In acknowledgement of these connections, I hereafter refer to what is interchangeably described as the medical, biomedical (Engel 1977) or technocratic model (Davis-Floyd 1992, 1994) as the techno-medical model; a term used by Oakley (1986). This emphasises ideological alliance between medicine, technology and capitalism, with medical technological 'progress' being continually fuelled by the enormous vested interests of the multinational corporations; for example the pharmaceutical, medical equipment and infant formula companies.

## Scientification of medicine

The scientific assumptions of the Enlightenment powerfully influenced the practice of medicine. Two major influences upon medicine were reductionism and dualism, concepts referred to earlier. The combination of reductionism and dualism when applied to medicine enabled the patient to be conceptually separated into mind, body and soul, with the body seen, like a machine, as something which could be taken apart, examined and repaired (Davis-Floyd 1994). As Illich observes, it was a philosophy which:

> effectively turned the human body into clock works and placed a new distance, not only between soul and body, but also between the patient's complaint and the physician's eye. Within this mechanised framework, pain turned into a red light and sickness into mechanical trouble.
>
> (Illich 1995: 160)

Within this reductionist and separatist model, the medical practitioner came to be seen as a grand mechanic or engineer, the caretaker of the body and its component parts (Schwarz 1990; Davis-Floyd and St John 1998). As Doyal and Pennell (1979) state, the separatist ideology extended to the practitioner and patient, requiring the doctor, as if a natural scientist, to separate himself from the subject as the scientist does from the natural world. In this way, scientific medicine became 'curative, individualistic and interventionist, objectifying patients and denying their status as social beings' (Doyal and Pennell 1979: 30).

The effects of reductionism and dualism on the recipients of medicine are also referred to by Doyal and Pennell (1979):

> The belief that one's mind and body can be separated and treated according to the laws of science, both serve to emphasise the loss of individual autonomy and the feelings of powerlessness so common in other areas of social and economic life.
>
> (Doyal and Pennell 1979: 43)

Stacey (1997) describes this sense of ontological separation in her reflexive account of a personal experience of developing cancer. She describes the ways in which she felt she became little more than the owner of a growth, with medical emphasis focusing upon concreteness, visibility, physicality and progress and presenting her disease as statistical, quantifiable and observable.

## Establishment of the hospital

Doyal and Pennell (1979) refer to the mass movement of people during the Industrial Revolution into rapidly expanding cities. The working classes and their families were exposed to damp, unsanitary housing, with overcrowding, infections, inadequate nutrition and lack of sunlight. These conditions contributed to the formation of a multiple range of diseases and bone deformities. The profoundly unhealthy nature of cities during the late eighteenth and early nineteenth centuries paved the way for the establishment of large hospitals for the sick. The hospital thus represented the place and space in which the principles underpinning techno-medicine flourished, with the scene set for a growing power base for medical doctors.

The discovery of disease as an identifiable entity through germ theory during the late nineteenth century, and the development of microscopy and related diagnostic techniques, reinforced the authority of medicine and the power of the doctor (Apple 1987; Lupton 1994). In the hospital, doctors were able to increasingly utilise the tools of their trade to diagnose, classify and treat disease. As Apple notes:

> New diagnostic tools unveiled to the physician but not the patient, the hidden mysteries of the human body. In providing the physicians with information not directly available to the patient, these instruments accentuated the esoteric nature of medical-scientific knowledge, thereby altering the doctor–patient relationship and strengthening the authority of the physician.
>
> (Apple 1987: 17)

Ill health within cities was seen as justification for the needs of the growth of institutional medicine. The poor inevitably welcomed the provision of free medical care through the hospital forum (Doyal and Pennell 1979; Apple 1987; Lewis 1980, 1990) and, like doctors, increasingly viewed science as progress and a symbol of medical authority (Apple 1987; Lupton 1994). Public health legislation, and subsequent initiatives such as improvements to the quality of water and sewage disposal, occurred concurrently but independently to techno-medicine (Doyal and Pennell 1979; Tew 1995). These had a major impact upon health from the late nineteenth century onwards but it was, and still is, commonly scientifically based medicine that took the credit. This set the scene for the ongoing further proliferation of techno-medicine. By the twentieth century, medical knowledge had gained supreme authoritative status through its inextricable links with prediction and control, and prevention of the eruption of disease, uncertainty and chaos (Engel 1977; Doyal and Pennell 1979; Arney 1982; Apple 1987; Lupton 1994). The powerful socialising effects of hospital medicine, as Illich (1995) argues, constructed a population of consumers of this commodity, for 'when cities are built around vehicles, they devalue human feet' (42).

The perspective of Foucault (1977) is of considerable relevance to this thesis in that he focuses upon the development of the hospital and the associated institution of medicine as an 'examining apparatus' (185). He asserts that the model of the Panopticon was employed to enable the development of specific hierarchies, spatial arrangements and surveillance systems centred around the requirement to make visible and supervise activities (Foucault 1977, 1980). Hospitals became places where patients could be observed, separated and supervised to prevent the spread of disease. The Nightingale wards with their two rows of patients separated by a central walkway facilitated this separation and scrutiny (Street 1992).

Foucault (1980) describes the hospital as a 'fragment of space closed in upon itself, a place of internment', a place characterised by scrupulously imposed spatial order, while concomitantly conveying the 'incessant disorder of comings and goings', 'inefficient medical surveillance' and inadequate achievement of its objective to improve health (177–178). He further comments:

> The space of the hospital must be organised according to a certain therapeutic strategy, through the uninterrupted presence and hierarchical prerogatives of doctors, through systems of observation, notation and record-taking which make it possible to fix the knowledge of different cases, to follow their particular evolution.
>
> (Foucault 1980: 180)

Foucault (1977, 1976, 1981) refers to normalising judgement within hospitals; rituals and techniques which established a power of normalisation over individuals. For Foucault (1977) the normal was established in standardised trainings; for example the national medical profession and through hospital systems. These trainings and systems were capable of operating general norms of health and a level of standardisation seen in industrial processes and products. Normalisation is seen in 'the case' and the way in which it is described, judged, measured, compared with others (191). Foucault (1981) emphasises the power of medicine through its techniques of questioning, monitoring, watching, spying, searching out, palpating and bringing into the light to label what is normal and what is deviant. Thus medicine socially constructs reality through its power to define what constitutes normality and therefore abnormality (deviance). Surveillance also extended to the body through the medical 'gaze' during the clinical encounter. This form of surveillance inscribes the body to such an extent that the individual starts to police or self-monitor her/his own body (Foucault 1976; 1980, Lupton 1994; Ribbens 1998). The concept of the medical gaze has now extended to a general increase in surveillance of the population by the state in the form of public health; for example child health clinics and medicine (Foucault 1976; Doyal and Pennell 1979; Lawler 1991; Lupton 1994,1995). Illich (1995) extends this notion in referring to society as having become a clinic overseeing and regulating people's health to ensure that they remain within normal limits.

## Techno-medical (re)production

### Technologising birth

A most striking example of the impact of the scientification of medicine and the establishment of the hospital may be seen in relation to women's (re)productive health in western countries such as the UK and US. As the medicalisation of life and the conceptualisation of the body as a machine were largely male-led, the idealised machine was seen as that of the man. Deviations from this prototype were represented in the female body that came to be seen as dysfunctional (Ehrenreich and English 1979; Martin 1987; Davis-Floyd 1992, 1994). This view contributed in part to changing the face of the birth experience for women.

From the seventeenth century onwards, an inexorable rise of the male obstetrician was accompanied by a diminishing definition of normality and an erosion of the midwife's domain (Ehrenreich and English 1979; Arney 1982; Kirkham 1983; Oakley 1986; Goer 1995; Tew 1995). Pregnancy and birth were gradually reconstituted and redefined from a social aspect of women's lives to a biomedical event prone to failure, danger and unpredictability and therefore requiring medical supervision and management (Oakley 1986; Schwarz 1990; Kohler Reissman 1992; Davis-Floyd 1992, 1994; Duden 1993). Franklin (1991) notes, in relation to the displacement of the social model with the biological one:

> the awesome measure of the power of medico-scientific discourse that it can accomplish this simultaneous erasure and replacement of something so basic to human social life as reproduction, through the power of its exclusive claim to represent the truth of 'natural facts'.
>
> (Franklin 1991: 200)

During the course of a single century, hospital replaced the home as the place and space in which women gave birth and recovered postnatally. In the UK, for example, hospital birth rates rose to over 60 per cent by the 1950s and by the 1990s, 98 per cent of women were birthing in NHS hospitals (Tew 1995). Hospitalisation of birth contributed to an undermining of women's knowledge about childbearing by isolating it from the community. In this way, women's knowledge generated from their embodied experiences came to be 'superseded', 'delegitimised', 'cognitively suppressed' and 'behaviourally managed' (Jordan 1997: 64).

The success of the techno-medical model of reproduction is complex and relates to several key issues. There was growing government concern, and accompanying recommendations regarding infant mortality and morbidity (Doyal and Pennell 1979). The material conditions of women's lives, and the powerfully persuasive lure of the hospital as the safe space and place in which to birth, contributed to women making demands for hospital births (Doyal and Pennell 1979; Lewis 1990). As Lewis (1990) notes, during the early twentieth century, women's groups such as the Women's Co-operative Guild, the Women's Labour League and the Fabian Women's Group campaigned actively for the pain relief and 'safety' offered by hospital births. Working-class women saw hospital birth and postnatal recovery as a welcome respite from damp, overcrowded, unsanitary living conditions and the profound exhaustion from repeated pregnancies, caring for a large family and exploitative paid working conditions (Llewelyn Davies 1978; Doyal and Pennell 1979; Lewis 1980, 1990). Lewis (1990) states:

What is clear is that women of all social classes in the early twentieth century expressed fear of childbirth in terms of both the pain and the considerable chance of subsequent health problems. Their fears were real and arose directly from the conditions of maternity they experienced. When these are understood, their demand for hospital births becomes readily comprehensible.

(Lewis 1990: 20)

Nevertheless, as Lewis (1990) asserts, women bought into a system in which medical domination and its accompanying 'technological sophistication' came to wield an authority through the hospitals and a momentum that became very difficult to challenge or reverse (26). Martin (1987) highlights the hegemonic connections between the ensuing hospitalisation of women when in labour and birth, and industrialisation. Based on interviews with women about their experiences of labour and birth she extends the metaphor of a woman's body as machine and medics as mechanics. She argues that with the development of hospitalised, complex management of birth, women have come to be seen as part of an industrial factory. In this portrayal, labour is a production process, the woman is the labourer, her uterus is the machine, her baby is the product and the doctor is the factory supervisor or even owner. Although the midwife does not feature in Martin's text, she fits in well in this scenario as the 'shop floor worker' following the supervisor's instructions, as described by Kirkham (1989: 132).

As Davis-Floyd (1992) argues, this supports the assumptions that technocratic society, with the doctor as its representative, is the producer of the product, the baby, and through a series of symbolic rituals this becomes imposed upon the minds of women. Martin (1987) draws similar conclusions but frames her analysis within Marxist notions of man's alienation and separation from the product of his labour. She argues that, in accordance with this model, the labouring woman is likewise disconnected from her birth, seeing it as something that is managed and controlled by the system. Women thus represented themselves as 'fragmented – lacking a sense of autonomy in the world and feeling carried along by forces beyond their control' (Martin 1987: 194). Thus, she asserts, women come to see their bodies as defined by the implicit scientific metaphors that assume that 'women's bodies are engaged in "production" with the separation this entails (given our conception of production) between labourer and labourer, labourer and product, labourer and labour, and manager and labourer' (194).

Martin's much-quoted research took place in the era when active management of labour was advocated. This concept was first described in a widely circulated book authored by O'Driscoll et al. in 1980 with two subsequent editions being published in 1986 and 1993 (O'Driscoll et al. 1993). This approach centres upon obstetric involvement in all aspects of women's labour and birth: precise timing and measurement to monitor progress, and early acceleration of 'labour' when not progressing according to strict medical criteria. This model for managing women's labour and birth is closely aligned to the industrial model exemplified in a car factory and referred to as Fordism (Beynon 1973). Walsh elaborates on the similarities:

Both arrange activity around dissembled stages and with clear demarcations for employees' roles. As a car is 'birthed' following linear and discrete processes on an assembly line, so labouring women are processed through 'stages' using a mechanistic model. Both have a timescale for completion of product, and both have a highly sophisticated regulatory framework.

(Walsh 2006)

Several years after Martin's (1987) research, Davis-Floyd (1992) interviewed 100 American, middle-class women about their perceptions of birth. She found that almost half of the women saw themselves not as being controlled by technocracy, but as controlling and indeed manipulating the resources available to achieve their own requirements in birth. These women placed an enormous emphasis upon personal control and viewed their bodies as separate and indeed as serving them. Thus they had adopted a split mind–body view. The women saw modern birth facilities as empowering them to control an otherwise unpredictable biological experience. These women demonstrated 'conceptual fusion' with 'cognitive ease' with the techno-medical model and had come to see separateness and technology as normal and beneficial (Davis-Floyd 1992: 239). This highlights the strong socialising power of the hegemonic techno-medical model.

Arney (1982) highlights the increasing dependency upon 'monitoring, surveillance and normalisation' as the twentieth century progressed (8). The fetus became the second patient whose safety was placed in the hands of obstetricians, further legitimating a range of interventions. Thus Arney asserts 'the health of the baby, loaded with positive meanings for both mother and physician, justified continued active intervention in childbirth' (137). While the fetus grew in importance both literally and metaphorically, a concurrent compromise of feminine ontology occurred. As Blum (1999) states, in regard to erasure of the maternal body, 'for the disembodied mother, her body is not her own – but more than that, she is treated, and pressed to treat herself, as if body-less' (60).

The experience for women of surveillance and an intrusive dependency on visualisation is highlighted by Duden (1993) as one far removed from nurturing her unborn baby as a 'mystery' and 'hope', into one of being a vehicle for an endangered, increasingly visible fetus growing within the maternal 'ecosystem'. She highlights the metaphorical 'skinning' and 'disembodiment' of woman, so that she serves a 'nine month clientage' in which her 'scientifically' defined needs for help and counsel are addressed by professionals (4). This, she argues, necessitates dependency upon visual data that demystifies pregnancy and overrides sensations experienced by the woman. The mechanistic interpretations of such material place doctors in control of the information and establish abstract information as the defining element of pregnancy.

Surveillance extended beyond the mother and her baby to those providing the service, as noted above with reference to Foucault's (1977, 1980) discussion of Panopticism. As Arney (1982) states, 'monitoring is the new order of obstetrical control to which not only women and their pregnancies are subject but to which obstetrical personnel themselves are subject' (102). Thus a system was generated which insidiously encouraged conformity to the techno-medical norms through a complex combination of socialisation and surveillance. While there was resistance to the technologising of birth throughout the twentieth century by women's groups, non-governmental organisations and groups of midwives (Lewis 1980, 1990; Oakley 1986; Foley 1998; Edwards 2000, 2001, 2005), the general global trend continues towards maintenance and continuation of the techno-medical model of (re)production. The rising Caesarean section rates across the world to about 20 per cent of births provide a crucial indicator that societal fusion with this model persists and indeed grows (Johanson *et al.* 2002).

### Timing (re)production

The mechanical clock played an increasingly profound role in women's (re)productive experiences. As Forman and Sowton (1989) state, 'the insatiable urge of scientists and their technologies to quantify and impose linearity on the life cycle is nowhere more vividly seen than in male-dominated obstetrics' (xiii). Over the course of the twentieth century, in parallel with increasing hospitalisation, every aspect of women's (re)productive experience became increasingly viewed through the tyrannical lens of linear time (Fox 1989; Kahn 1989; Pizzini 1992; Thomas 1992; Davis-Floyd 1992, 1994; Edwards 2001, 2005; Simonds 2002). Thus, as Fox (1989) argues, by substituting a male model of productivity for the archetype of the creative and transformative mother, obstetrics turned birth into a mechanical act and a time-bounded process. The pervasive effects of time on women's labouring bodies are emphasised by Thomas (1992):

> Time provides not only a way of describing the distribution of events but also a basis for interpretations and explanations. In reproduction it provides a way of distinguishing between normal and the abnormal, between the abnormal and the pathological. More generally this can be seen as a differentiation of the ordered from the disordered, the orderly from the disorderly.
>
> (Thomas 1992: 65)

While linear time now permeates many aspects of women's (re)productive experiences, we see an exponential increase in its oppressive potential as labour progresses and reaches its climax, the birth. A recent discourse analysis of selected obstetric and midwifery texts conducted by Simonds (2002) illustrates well the tyranny of obstetric timings. She states that 'obstetrics works on women's bodies to make them stay on time and on course' with the discourse of obstetrics managing pregnancy and birth by 'institutionalising rigid time standards, carving procreative time up into increasingly fragmented units, which are imbued with the potential for danger' (559, 560). Simonds (2002) further asserts that in obstetric management, 'interventions have become more common, the notion that obstetrics can – and should – work against the bodily clock that stops too soon or continues too long has gained credence (563) and furthermore, 'in obstetrics, time signifies the danger unmanaged women's bodies represent. Now women are bound by the clock rather than leather straps' (568).

Simonds (2002) contrasts this notion of time seen in a classic obstetric text, *Williams Obstetrics* (from 1971–1997) (Cunningham *et al.* 1993), with that seen in Ina May Gaskin's (1990) well-known text, *Spiritual Midwifery*. Recognising these as ideological poles, she asserts that *Spiritual Midwifery* exemplifies an 'essentialist orthodoxy wholly antithetical to medicalized environments and, thus, to prevalent cultural ideology about procreative events' (569). The obstetric text centres on women labouring against time while Gaskin's text focuses upon women being active in time, with indeed the focus moving clearly away from any notion of time constraint. Simonds (1992) states in relation to Gaskin's text:

> Time is not something to be rationed; not a scarce commodity that procreating women waste; not a route toward measuring pathology nor, in itself, an indication of pathology; not a series of obstacles against which women's performance must be measured; and not a means of industrialising the labour process. Time just *is*. Birthing women can take their time, rather than have it taken from them.
>
> (Simonds 1992: 569)

As women's experiences of (re)production were reconstituted and reconfigured by Enlightenment thought, so were their experiences of child-rearing, which also became part of women's productive projects, and to which I now turn.

## Production of people to function in society

Preoccupation with industrial production for profit, eugenicist government concerns to produce sufficient quantities of future citizens to 'man' armies and industry, and the super-valuation of rationalistic science, pervasively and powerfully influenced child 'care' practices across many western countries during the Enlightenment period. Although production in the industrial and economic sense was ascribed largely as a matter for men, women in the designated (re)productive role were inextricably linked with production of the next generation. As Lupton (1996) states, 'mothers domesticate children, propelling them from the creature of pure instinct and uncontrolled wildness of infancy into the civility and self-regulation of adulthood' (39).

Beekman (1977) discusses, in his historical analysis of child-rearing practices over the centuries, the role of the 'good' mother in taming babies and preparing them for the requirements of, and scrutiny by, society. He highlights the parental project of creating and adapting children to society's demands whilst simultaneously protecting them from society's ills. Consequently child 'care' advice has 'reflected the nature of society and morality in a given historical period' (xiii). Likewise, science and medicine not only infiltrated women's experiences of pregnancy and birth, but also became central in defining motherhood. As Miller (1998) states, 'transition to motherhood is surrounded by pervasive ideologies – both biologically determined and socially constructed which can be clearly discerned before and long after a child is born' (58).

It is crucial at this point to make it clear that we cannot simply see parenting advice and practices as being imposed upon women without regard to the complex socio-economic and cultural influences at play. Women were themselves socialised through society and exposed to the values and imperatives of the times. They participated in dissemination of the current contemporary thoughts on childcare through women's groups and related publications (Lewis 1980, 1990; Apple 1987; Carter 1995; Blum 1999). The material conditions of women's lives likewise influenced childcare; for example a working-class family would necessarily become engaged in 'producing' children capable of early independence and paid employment as a means of survival for the family. Nevertheless, the pervasive influence of dominant ideologies should not be underestimated.

The works of Foucault (1977, 1981) and Beekman (1977) illuminate a central imperative emerging from the Enlightenment period onwards, reaching a peak during the nineteenth century: the requirement to mould individuals for the rigours of the factory. A growing obsession developed with authority, discipline, obedience and endeavours to rid a child of bad habits such as manifestations of an emerging sexuality, self-love and self-indulgence (Beekman 1977; Foucault 1981). A concurrent preoccupation with clocks, routines and schedules, again related to the requirements of efficient factory production, meant that the baby could be disciplined by the clock. The progressive urbanisation of societies with the accompanying social isolation and rootlessness meant that women increasingly sought and engaged with sources of 'expert advice' in place of intergenerational and embodied knowledges.

Beekman (1977) argues that by the twentieth century there was a 'conscious, systematic effort to actually turn the child into a biological machine' (110):

> Little was known about children in a scientific sense but a good deal was known about production. Production demanded regularity, repetition and scheduling. All that seemed to be required of the family was that the parents submit to the kind of systematization and discipline in the handling of their children as was routinely required of factory workers on a production line.
>
> (Beekman 1977: 113)

Although very little was known about children, this era marked the proliferation of scientific/medical dogma and advice related to children across many western countries (Beekman 1977). From the late nineteenth and early twentieth centuries, as Apple (1987) argues, scientific motherhood was culturally constructed and emerged as a 'coherent ideology' (97). While women were defined as essentially maternal they were increasingly exhorted to pay regard to scientific and medical expertise. This related in part to western governments' concerns that high levels of infant mortality were detrimental in terms of production of men for the army and industries (Doyal and Pennell 1979). This opened the door to a wide range of state interference ranging from education of mothers to comprehensive surveillance through, for example, welfare clinics and health visiting (Doyal and Pennell 1979; Oakley 1986; Apple 1987; Lupton 1994; Carter 1995). These were carried out with 'little regard for the material circumstances generated by the inequalities within the capitalist economy' (Doyal and Pennell 1979: 164). An entire industry developed around mothering and baby care. As Apple (1987) describes, baby books and magazines started to flourish from the early twentieth century, covering matters such as infant feeding, hygiene and toileting. Advertising in these magazines emphasised the importance of taking professional advice in choosing products, each advocating their own scientific and medically endorsed background.

The obsession with controlling the baby's behaviour, combined with the super-valuation of objective rationalistic science, reached its zenith when behavioural psychology came into vogue in the 1920s. As Beekman (1977) illustrates, it was during this period that institutional attitudes most powerfully infiltrated the home. The baby was considered to be a blank slate (tabula rasa) and mother and child were expected to be 'separate' both physically and emotionally, with love seen as corrupting. The child was to be taught self-control, routine and discipline with mothers avoiding playing, rocking, cuddling and any form of sensuous activity. Activities of the child were observed, measured, recorded, analysed and all compared to standards being set with increasing authority. Blum (1999) asserts that the behaviourists reshaped the norms of embodied attachment, as they warned mothers against being over-solicitous or rewarding bad behaviour, for example crying, by rocking or cuddling the baby. This, she states, was the era of rational discipline, habit training and measured love, all under medical supervision.

From the 1930s, as Beekman (1977) notes, society was in a state of flux and the economy in a state of collapse. Scientific ideas related to parenting and children likewise began to be challenged and changed. This led to a gradual emergence in some circles of an emphasis upon emotional interaction between mother and baby and a recognition that the mother should make allowance for the child as guide-in-part to her/his needs. The concept of demand feeding emerging in the 1940s, to which I return later, constitutes an example of changing attitudes. Beekman (1977) associates the softening of attitudes with changing views regarding the individual being the mainstay of democracy, and changes in societal views evolving during the two world wars. Nazi authoritarianism, for example, caused a major questioning about the desire for parents to exert absolute authority over their children.

It is important to recognise that although trends in childcare changed, there was not a mighty sweep across society. Throughout the remainder of the twentieth century, and into the twenty-first century, ideologies around 'natural' and baby/child-led approaches have been juxtaposed with counter-arguments. A classical example may be seen in the current upsurge of 'authoritative' texts arguing for a return to the disciplined approaches of the early twentieth century. The recent book by Ford (1999), *The Contented Baby Book,* speaks volumes about these contradictory trends. Ford advocates a return to management of the baby using hour-by-hour, day-by-day routines, representing a re-emphasis upon timings, precision, control and separation. Whichever philosophy of parenting women adopt in contemporary western society, they are still expected to civilise their baby, with food and eating being key routes to achieving this (Lupton 1996; Schmied 1998). This overview of the ways in which the values of society influence parenting therefore sets the scene for my focus upon infant feeding practices in Chapter 2.

# Chapter 2

# Formulating infant feeding

## Introduction

In this chapter, I discuss critical moments of significance that have influenced infant feeding and, more specifically, breastfeeding policy and practice in industrialised countries across the world. This includes discussion around the medicalisation of infant feeding and the marketing of breast-milk substitutes. The hospital is highlighted as the place in which breastfeeding became institutionally regulated and notions of how to feed infants became ideologically pervasive. I also focus upon breastfeeding within the fabric of women's lives, acknowledging that there are multiple and complex influences upon their infant feeding decisions and experiences.

## The influences of Enlightenment thought

Changes in infant feeding practices from the Enlightenment to the twenty-first century represent a powerful illustration of the highly complex interaction between dominant ideologies, commerce and women's lives. Enlightenment principles had a profound impact upon subsequent infant feeding practices. However, breastfeeding cannot be seen as a 'simple' activity that was conducted exclusively by all mothers until utterly disrupted by science and medicine. While techno-medicine and commercialisation have indeed contributed to a striking disruption of breastfeeding and a dramatic loss of intergenerational, community-based knowledge, this needs to be viewed in connection with the socio-cultural context of women's lives; this is an issue I return to later. While I acknowledge that there has been considerable hegemonic enculturation of women in this area, as Apple (1987) argues, women actively engaged with, and participated in, infant feeding practice changes during the past century, with the feminist movement playing a substantial role.

Historical (Fildes 1986) and anthropological literature (Maher 1992a; Dettwyler 1995; Wiessinger 1995; Vincent 1999) make it clear that the global history of infant feeding is very complex, with women supplementing breast milk with a range of alternative, symbolic foods, often from a very early age. Practices were highly varied, as influenced by prevailing socio-economic systems, cultural beliefs about the role of women as mothers, and the material conditions of women's lives. As Carter (1995) states, 'many of the building blocks of current discourses have been moulded over centuries. The changing "fashions" of infant feeding are frequently expressions of the way in which nature, culture and science are conceptualised within any particular period' (35).

Enlightenment thought profoundly influenced attitudes to infant feeding in western industrialised countries. Towards the end of the nineteenth century and into the twentieth century there was growing scientific, medical and governmental interest and involvement in infant feeding practices. Prior to this era, infant feeding was largely the domain of women. Both public policy and medical recommendations were related to concerns regarding high rates of infant mortality and the quality of the population (Doyal and Pennell 1979; Lewis 1980; Carter 1995). As Doyal and Pennell (1979) note, this agenda was driven by the need for industrialised countries to provide plentiful 'fit' individuals to engage in the various forms of production. The behaviour of the mother was consequently scrutinised and called into question at all stages of ongoing policy decision-making (Fildes 1986; Carter 1995).

One of the first major areas of debate and subsequent influence appears to be upon the practice of wet nursing, a key way in which women engaged either significant others or paid employees to nurture their babies when they were unavailable or indisposed (Fildes 1986). The medical profession increasingly discredited this practice during the nineteenth century. They expressed concerns about its biological, social and moral shortcomings, so that by the twentieth century wet nursing was virtually non-existent in western communities (Apple 1987; Fildes 1986; Ebrahim 1991; Palmer 1993). Apple (1987) notes that during the same period the quality of the mother's milk or feeding practices came to be scientifically questioned. Although breast milk was considered to be natural and ideal, it was proclaimed that not all women could produce enough or adequate milk, with a growing list of medical reasons being put forward (Apple 1987; Wolf 2000). As Wolf (2000) states, 'the notion that human lactation is an unreliable body function became a cultural truth that has persisted unabated to the present day' (93).

The scientific discourses around infant feeding at the turn of the twentieth century (Rotch 1890; Budin 1907; Vincent 1910; King 1913) reflected the mechanistic, dualistic and reductionist assumptions of the Enlightenment. They also reflected the growing medical imperative to supervise and regulate women's bodies and minimise the threat of chaos (Palmer 1993; Carter 1995; Blum 1999; Smale 2000). Metaphors used presented breast milk as a disembodied product, produced in a mechanical way as in a classical factory of the times. The woman was rendered invisible, unless there were problems that she was then blamed for.

A paper obtained from the Royal Society of Medicine, London, authored by Thomas Rotch (1890) entitled 'The management of human breast-milk in cases of difficult infantile digestion' illustrates the application of the techno-medical model to medical advice on infant feeding. Rotch was Professor of the diseases of children, Harvard University; Physician to the Infants' Hospital, Boston; and Consulting Physician to the Infants' Hospital, London. His work was highly regarded on both sides of the Atlantic and indeed Ralph Vincent, senior physician to the Infants' Hospital, Westminster, dedicated his text book *The Nutrition of the Infant* (1910) to Rotch 'in acknowledgement of his scientific achievements' (vi). The context for the paper by Rotch (1890) is clearly that of the industrial production process, with the dominant metaphor being the factory, in this case a mill, as highlighted in the statement:

> The breasts of all mammals that suckle their young, are elaborators, producers; they are not storehouses for preserving sustenance for the infant until it is needed; they are beautifully-constructed mills, turning out when demand is made for it, a product which has been directly moulded within their walls, from the material which has been brought to it and through its portals from various parts of the economy.
>
> (Rotch 1890: 89)

The baby is clearly the consumer of the product: 'This delicate mechanism adapts itself as to the bulk of its product, elaborating a smaller or greater supply according to the age and again the size of the consumer' (89). The breasts in several places are referred to as machinery: 'This machinery is regulated as to the time which it is required at different ages of the consumer to produce the average qualitative food' (90). The breasts appear to be viewed by Rotch as potentially defective in that the constituents and/or volume are easily disturbed and rendered incorrect:

> The epithelial cells are so finely organised, so sensitive with minute nerve connections, that changes of atmosphere, changes in food, the emotions, fatigue, sickness, the catamenia, pregnancy, and many influences, in fact, throw their mechanism out of gear most readily, and change essentially the proportions of their finished product.
>
> (Rotch 1890: 89)

Here the female body is once again represented as a machine that is unpredictable and prone to inefficiency and malfunction. The mother is largely invisible from the twelve-page paper by Rotch (1890), being rarely mentioned in comparison to numerous references to 'the breasts' and 'the baby'. The dualistic language clearly compartmentalises the parts of the body and separates them from the person. The text contains repeated reference to the breasts without reference to the mother. In one place, when she is referred to in association with her breasts, she is simply referred to as an organism, 'The mechanism of the mammary gland, therefore, is in its most perfect condition after the colostrum period has ceased, and when the general organism, both physical and mental is in a state of rest' (91). This rendering of the mother as invisible is raised in a number of other critical studies related to pregnancy and childbirth (Oakley 1986; Martin 1987; Duden 1993), but is little discussed in relation to her breastfeeding.

There is frequent reference by Rotch (1890) to the quantities of particular substances and minute breakdown of breast-milk substances. The specific quantities of named nutrients, for example albuminoids, are attributed to the woman's diet, temperament and lifestyle and are seen as correctable: 'A sedentary life, with abundance of rich food (provided the woman has a strong healthy digestion) appears to increase the total solids and decrease the water' (94). Several tables show the constituents of milk and refer to 'normal milk', 'poor milk', 'over rich milk' and 'bad milk' (95).

On the occasions in which Rotch (1890) refers to the mother it is in the context of her diet, temperament and behaviour and its influence upon the milk's constituents. Advice is then given as to how to increase specific constituents in the milk; for example 'a meat or rather nitrogenous diet in the woman increases the fat in her milk' (94). Temperament/mental state is blamed for 'throwing their [breast cells] mechanism out of gear most readily and changing essentially the proportions of their finished product' (89). Behaviour is scrutinised; for example the mother is blamed for neglecting to time feed intervals correctly, which results in 'qualitative changes' in the milk (90). The woman's behaviour is clearly seen to be in need of regulation to ensure that the milk is of the right quality and quantity; for example:

> It is physical exercise which we must insist on, preferably walking in the open air, and within the limits of fatigue. An average of from one to two miles twice daily I have found to be about what the average healthy woman needs to reduce her albuminoid per centage.
>
> (Rotch 1890: 95)

The breasts appear to be seen by Rotch (1890) as in need of 'management' seemingly independently of their owners! For example; 'I have a large number of breasts, in private practice especially, but also in the hospitals, pumped for analysis' (96). Breast milk itself is seen as in need of management; for example table VI 'shows a bad milk, and one which was impossible to manage on account of the continual recurrence of the same cause, uncontrolled emotions' (96). Here we see the linking of the above themes of constituents and the mother's temperament and how this may or may not be managed. Another illustration is seen in relation to table X headed, 'Shows the value of retaining the breast-milk by managing even an unpromising case' (98). It is stated, 'The above represents a bad milk from the failure of the healthy mother to conform to the rules of lactation' (98). This is followed by a meticulously precise description of the incremental improvements in the milk achieved by prescriptive management of the mother in terms of her mental state, pumping of her breast, one mile of exercise and eating more meat.

In summary, the paper by Rotch (1890) exemplifies the techno-medical approach, being worded in authoritative manner, rendering the woman's breasts and breast milk as disembodied from her person, and managed as a production process along the highly regimented lines of the factories in existence at the turn of the century. The tone is paternalistic, with the mother being referred to only in terms of her correct or incorrect behaviour as dictated by male experts.

Within other early texts about infant feeding (Rotch 1890; Budin 1907; Vincent 1910; King 1913) this fear of chaos and desire to control is highly consistent; for example:

> In all cases the success or failure of maternal nursing must largely depend upon the way in which the practical details are carried out. Where the methods are haphazard, and the mother feeds her infant at all sorts of times, sometimes over feeding and at other times underfeeding it, the results are always unsatisfactory, and the infant is constantly suffering from digestive disturbance in some form; while in other cases the effects are much more serious. Twelve hours after the birth the infant should be put to the breast and allowed to suck for two or three minutes. From this time to the time that the breasts are freely supplying milk, the infant should be given the breast every four hours [...]. It is a serious mistake to allow the infant to take freely of the colostrum when this is plentiful. In anything but a small amount, colostrum seriously disturbs the infant – a fact that is not at all surprising when its chemical constitution is considered.
>
> (Vincent 1910: 40)

The mother is again rendered almost invisible in this scenario, as her breasts are discussed as if independent of the owner, except to comment on her failure to follow practical details. The reader is then referred to a table of feed frequencies, commencing with the first day and continuing for four to six months, with one feed a night permitted until the infant is twelve weeks old, when it should be discontinued. Medical anxiety is expressed regarding the initial weight loss, with test-weighing becoming a part of the ritual, i.e. weighing before and after a feed in order to calculate the amount of milk taken and routine weighing also being developed as a means of ensuring that the correct amounts were taken. Later regimes also dictated that feeds should be meticulously and rigidly controlled in terms of time spent at each breast measured to the nearest minute; for example two minutes per breast per feed on the first day, five minutes on the second day, seven minutes on the third, ten minutes on the fourth, and from then on twenty minutes maximum on each breast (Fisher 1985). This led to the baby being deprived of mother's fat-rich hind milk creating a hungry dissatisfied baby and had the potential to lead to a secondary milk insufficiency and a generally negative experience for the mother (Fisher 1985; Woolridge 1995). In this way, milk insufficiency becomes an embodied reality.

## The hospital as centre stage for 'scientific' feeding

The twentieth century brought with it the dramatic increase in hospitalisation of women during childbirth and postnatal recovery, as stated. This provided a system in which implementation of practices in line with Enlightenment thought could flourish (Carter 1995). The hospital was the place in which the principles of linear time, production, control and surveillance predominated. Scheduling and placing of rigid time controls upon every aspect of the breastfeeding relationship became central as the twentieth century progressed. This scheduling of breastfeeding provides a classic example of the imposition of time constraints upon an inherently cyclical, rhythmical and relational process. As Simonds (2002) states, the 'idiosyncratic rhythms of breastfeeding (determined by mothers and newborns) were obfuscated and mechanically regulated by an obsessively precise schedule' (566). Millard (1990) provides an excellent illustration of the ways in which the clock became central to medical ideology around infant feeding. She conducted a literary analysis of twentieth-century paediatric texts as manifestations of the formal system of biomedical knowledge in the US. She states, 'The clock has provided the main frame of reference, creating regimentation reminiscent of factory work, segmenting breastfeeding into a series of steps, and emphasising efficiency in time and motion' (211) and furthermore:

> The clock has an unparalleled position as a symbol of science, discipline, and the co-ordination of human effort. Its very use in formulating advice thus confers legitimacy on pediatric breastfeeding recommendations in the eyes of both lay women and physicians themselves. The cultural themes implicit in pediatric advice also connect to the clock – the factory model for physiological processes and social co-ordination, the ideal of flexible advice coupled with firm structuring, the ascendancy of professional advice in family matters and the necessity of regularity in maternal–infant interactions.
>
> (Millard 1990: 217)

Balsamo *et al.*'s (1992) research highlights the impact of this clock-controlled regimentation upon women. She interviewed forty women in their own homes regarding their experiences of breastfeeding following birthing in hospitals or clinics in Turin in the 1970s and 1980s. Women reported feeling alienated from their bodies and breastfeeding as they conformed to a factory like scheduling of their early mothering and breastfeeding experiences. Balsamo *et al.* (1992) refer to the ways in which paediatric scheduling of breastfeeding brought the mother into a type of time which related to efficiency and productivity derived from industrial/patriarchal society. The imposition of industrial time upon the experience of breastfeeding caused conflict for the women.

With growing hospitalisation came a strong emphasis upon hygiene and the combat of infection. Doctors, midwives and nurses wholeheartedly enforced anti-infection control. As Palmer (1993) describes, the ideas around hygiene also contributed to the development of nurseries and separation of babies from mothers for the duration of the hospital stay. The babies were attended to by masked nurses in the nurseries and brought to mothers for feeds only. Mothers were required to wear masks and cleansing of their nipples and breasts became routine. As Blum (1999) states, 'As hospitals sanitized and covered the mother's body and breasts and scrubbed her nipples, they conveyed that she and her baby were not to be trusted' (30). The postnatal ward geography facilitated surveillance and separation of mothers 'safe' distances apart to avoid spread of infection.

The combination of practices described above was highly detrimental to the establishment of breastfeeding, leaving women with a profound loss of confidence in their ability to breastfeed (Fisher 1985; Palmer 1993). The loss of confidence was further fuelled by the commercialisation of infant feeding, to which I now turn.

## The infant formula industry

The growth of the infant formula industry in western industrialised countries during the late nineteenth and early twentieth century occurred concurrently and symbiotically with the scientific and medical interest in breastfeeding. Palmer (1993) summarises the impetus for this growth during the late nineteenth century commencing with a scientific interest in the analysis of milk, human and animal, and its conversion into formula for administration via a feeding bottle. The dairy industry was at the same time becoming more efficient and low-cost cows' milk increased in availability. The availability of large quantities of surplus milk and the development of milk separation and drying processes encouraged the establishment of milk laboratories during the early twentieth century for production of dried formula milk. Developing techniques such as pasteurisation of milk led to what has been described as the 'clean milk movement' (Baumslag and Michels 1995: 120), providing further justification for the 'safe' humanisation of milk. The growth of the cheese industry created excess whey products that became increasingly expensive to transport or dispose of, so their use for infant formulae provided the ideal economic solution (Ebrahim 1991; Palmer 1993).

As the twentieth century progressed, the expanding multinational corporations increasingly used placards, posters and the growing media channels such as radio and television to market their products (Sokol 1997). Key advertising messages portrayed breastfeeding as prone to failure, unsophisticated, outmoded and primitive, whilst bottle feeding was being associated with western affluence, consumerism and the liberated woman (Jelliffe and Jelliffe 1978; Palmer 1993). In line with the capitalist and consumerist society, the bottle was incorporated with the advertising of high-status commodities such as fast cars and household luxuries (Baer 1982). The promotion of infant formula clearly located infant feeding within the discourses of production and consumerism, these concepts being central to the market economy.

The proliferation of healthcare facilities in western industrialised countries, such as maternity hospitals and child welfare clinics, and the increasing hospitalisation of women giving birth during the twentieth century, provided an ideal focus for the promotion of infant formula. As Palmer (1993) describes, a model of co-operation developed as formula companies and doctors became aware of their interdependence. The formula companies rapidly realised that marketing through healthcare facilities caused the public to perceive direct endorsement of the products by the health workers, and use of such channels enabled massive expansion of their sales. Consequently, they heavily courted medical staff, providing gifts and financial incentives to doctors and hospitals and directing their target consumer groups through doctors in order to obtain formula. As Apple (1987) remarks, the relationships that developed were mutually beneficial in that formula companies increasingly emphasised the importance of medical supervision in making up feeds and the feeding process in general. Doctors in turn endorsed the products that emphasised the importance of medical supervision as scientific and desirable. These two powerful groups, doctors and infant formula manufacturers, in turn influenced government policies.

Oakley (1986) connects the scientific interest in adapting animal milks with the growing infant welfare movement and, as part of that development, with milk dispensaries. These dispensaries originated in France in the 1890s and the idea took off in Britain and the US during the same decade. There were fifteen such depots in Britain by 1907, administered by public health authorities. The purpose was to provide reduced-cost, 'safe', 'humanised' milk and hygienic teats for mothers, with the poor being specifically targeted;

> The main principle of the milk depot was municipal control over the quality of milk from before it left the cow until the mother opened the municipally-supplied bottle to feed it to her infant. The milk depots thus aimed to cure one cause of maternal fecklessness, namely contaminated milk.
>
> (Oakley 1986: 39)

Oakley describes this 'safe milk movement' as the start of a 'systematic investment in the monitoring of maternal behaviour' which was extended to 'every crevice of the whole realm of housewifery and motherhood' (42). Carter (1995) refers to the payoff for the poor, in that if they attended for cheap milk they opened up themselves and their lives for public scrutiny. It was assumed that women should breastfeed, but if they had a good excuse not to they would be availed of suitable alternatives along with supervision. In the UK, these milk depots became infant welfare centres in 1915 (Carter 1995). The growing state and medical involvement in formula milks served to create the increasing sense that they were medicinal and desirable (Lewis 1980). This notion increased during the two world wars as the government invested in low-cost baby milks for mothers in an attempt to improve infant welfare (Carter 1995).

The global influence of formula companies expanded as the twentieth century progressed. They even became involved in the design of hospitals, which no doubt was intended to appear philanthropic. However, as Baer (1982) points out, the design is founded on the principle of maximum separation between mother and baby, with nurseries situated long distances from the mothers' beds. One of the most powerful marketing strategies involved the issue of free milk samples to health centres and hospitals. Company representatives dressed as milk nurses gave free samples directly to mothers when they visited and prior to discharge from hospital. This practice contributed towards the normalisation of infant formula and undermining of breastfeeding (Bergevin *et al.* 1983; Frank *et al.* 1987; Adair *et al.* 1993). Healthcare information on issues such as growth was displayed, with company and brand names, accompanied by potent messages suggesting that when breast milk was insufficient, infant formula was there to ensure optimum growth and health (Sokol 1997).

## Infant feeding trends and women's lives

From the end of the nineteenth century, infant feeding 'prescriptions' and practices fluctuated enormously. As the twentieth century progressed, within industrialised countries the option of providing infant formula to a baby became real, and although the general medical message centred upon breastfeeding as being the 'natural' and 'motherly' way to feed, there was a concomitant medical acknowledgement that not all mothers could 'manage' this and that there was a safe alternative available (Apple 1987; Carter 1995).

Carter's (1995) in-depth study of women who had babies between 1920 and 1980, in a city in the north-east of England, highlights the influences upon women's infant feeding decisions within an industrialised nation. She first makes the important point that many women breast *and* bottle feed, and each woman has her own complex, personal, socio-economic and intergenerational context. She conceptualises as 'working conditions' the situations in which infant feeding is practised, to avoid seeing breastfeeding as simply a biological activity. This, she argues, provides a 'disruptive reading of the dominant narrative of femininity' (79). She does, however, urge caution in this conceptualisation, in that it undervalues the relational aspect of infant feeding.

Carter's (1995) interviews revealed that for women in low socio-economic occupational groups there were clear barriers to prolonged and exclusive breastfeeding. These included unhealthy working conditions that were hazardous, time-consuming and exhausting. Housing was often cramped, with more than one generation co-existing. Breastfeeding became a symbol of poverty, associated with tough living conditions, large families, exhaustion, discomfort, embarrassment and restriction. Given the relentless demands upon women, Carter argues that bottle feeding provided women with some sense of control over their lives. It also enabled them to resist the exhortations to self-monitor their bodies and control aspects of their lives that were considered to affect their milk; for example their diet, emotions and exercise taken. This situation was also described by Apple (1987). The growing antipathy towards breastfeeding was compounded by reports of authoritarianism and lack of support in hospital combined with inadequate family support at home (Carter 1995).

Throughout the same period, women's groups that tended to have membership from higher socio-economic occupational groups were engaged in a socio-political movement to demand improved rights and conditions for women (Lewis 1980, 1990). As Blum (1999) notes, while they were more likely to subscribe to medical recommendations, middle-class women also saw breastfeeding as biologically tying. With the option of wet nursing removed, the bottle and infant formula came to be seen as a symbol of modernity, progress and a means to autonomy for affluent women. The clock and linear time were becoming rooted in the lives of women, as described above, and the precision, control and ability to measure infant formula was probably appealing. In contrast to women's socialisation into productive time, breastfeeding, as Carter (1995) notes, came to be seen as an activity conducted in women's own/private time.

Unique to the twentieth century was the sexual portrayal of women's breasts in industrialised countries through the growing media to sell commodities ranging from peanuts to fast cars and cigarettes (Palmer 1993). Breastfeeding, as stated, also came to be seen as associated with bodily fluids and therefore potentially 'dirty', contaminating and representative of the body being out of control (Bramwell 2001; Bartlett 2002). Consequently, while breastfeeding was commonly referred to as natural, it was becoming far from natural as a public activity, creating dissonance, embarrassment and anxiety to women from all social groupings (McConville 1994; Van Esterik 1994a; Rodriguez and Frazier 1995; Blum 1999).

The combination of the public–private divide that developed with growing industrialisation and the sexualisation of women's breasts led to breastfeeding becoming increasingly seen as a private activity to be conducted away from the public gaze (Maher 1992b; Carter 1995). However, as Carter (1995) notes, even in the so-called privacy of the woman's own home breastfeeding is not a neutral activity. Women wherever they were still had to negotiate 'what to do, where to do it, in whose presence, and with whose approval it can be done' (107). She states: 'What remained consistent was women's responsibility for being modest and discreet and checking out the implications of breastfeeding in each particular setting' (114).

Another constant throughout this period was the connection made by women's advocacy groups and the medical establishment that breastfeeding was the natural ideal with a discursive connection being made between mothering, breastfeeding and naturalness (Apple 1987; Leff *et al.* 1994; Carter 1995). This however created many difficulties for women. First, notions of natural as a cultural construction were, and are, ever changing, as Franklin (1997) states:

> Not only are constructions of the natural culturally and historically specific; they are also shifting and contradictory. As is the case in the analysis

of science, a cultural domain to which ideas of the natural are central, it is important not to overstate the discursive or cultural determinism operative in the 'naturalising' process.

(Franklin 1997: 97)

As discussed earlier, the 'natural ideal' was seen as prone to weakness and therefore in need of medical management. It was called into question by the general acknowledgement of the place for infant formula in a variety of circumstances. Equally, breastfeeding was becoming less visible as the sexual breast was growing in visibility. Given the living conditions for many women referred to above, as Carter (1995) reports, the notion of natural mothering and its associations became increasingly unappealing. In advocating breastfeeding as a natural ideal within a culture where this was increasingly no longer the norm, women's confidence was further eroded.

So, as the twentieth century progressed, women who carried out the deeply embodied experience of breastfeeding were required to engage increasingly in the negotiation of space in which they breastfed, the time in which it was conducted and the relationships with those around them. The combination of barriers and constraints to this negotiation process within the fabric of their daily lives, combined with increasing medicalisation of infant feeding and marketing of infant formula, led to the situation by the 1970s whereby, within three to four generations, women in industrialised countries around the world had turned from predominantly breastfeeding to largely formula feeding.

## Efforts to restore breastfeeding as the norm

I now focus upon international initiatives that endeavoured to restore, protect, promote and support breastfeeding as a practice. I first present a summary of UK government initiatives to illustrate one western industrialised country's attempt to 'turn the clock back'.

### UK government initiatives

By 1975, recordable breastfeeding rates had reached an all-time low in the UK. Ironically, this was the time when there was also a growing body of scientific research highlighting the nutritional and immunological benefits of breastfeeding for babies. In response to this paradox the UK government conducted and published a series of quinquennial infant feeding surveys that have continued into the twenty-first century (Martin 1978; Martin and Monk 1982; Martin and White 1988; White et al. 1992; Foster et al. 1997; Hamlyn et al. 2002). These reports documented breastfeeding initiation and continuation rates. They also charted infant feeding trends in relation to demographic variables, in particular social class and its correlates, such as levels of education beyond age eighteen, maternal age, and place where living.

These survey reports were used by the government to inform a series of policy documents (DHSS 1974, 1978, 1980, 1988a; DoH 1994). In the first such document it was acknowledged that the UK was largely an 'artificially fed nation' (DHSS 1974: 4). Later in the report, after a lengthy discussion about the problems associated with formula milk when compared to breast milk with regard to specific nutritional and anti-infective components, it was stated:

> We are convinced that satisfactory growth and development after birth is more certain when an infant is fed an adequate volume of breast milk, we recommend that all mothers be encouraged to breastfeed their babies for a minimum of two weeks and preferably for the first four to six months of life.
>
> (DHSS 1974: 24)

Between 1975 and 1980, the rates of women breastfeeding had increased quite markedly (see table). However, whilst those concerned with increasing rates may have seen the rise as reflective of their efforts, it seems more likely, as Woolridge (1994) suggests, that the change in women's practices reflected, particularly in the more highly educated sectors of the population, a return to whole foods and a healthier lifestyle. Blum (1999) refers to a similar trend in the US as the 'back to nature movement' (44). The breastfeeding rates in the UK thereafter have remained relatively static. Changes in sample characteristics from 1990 to 2000 render the small rises in rates between these years as even less significant than they appear to be.

In 1988, in response to concerns raised in the above reports and to the high discontinuation rates (DHSS 1988b), the government set up the Joint Breastfeeding Initiative. This group represented voluntary breastfeeding support groups and health professionals. It was replaced by the National Breastfeeding Working Group in 1992. The latter was led by a central co-ordinator and a network of health professionals across the UK, with a remit to act strategically to improve breastfeeding initiation and continuation rates. However, the paucity of government funding for these networks limited any major impact or effectiveness.

Percentage of women breastfeeding at birth, 6 weeks, and 4 months following the birth

|  | 1975 England and Wales | 1980 GB | 1985 GB | 1990 UK | 1995 UK | 2000 UK |
|---|---|---|---|---|---|---|
| Birth | 51 | 65 | 64 | 62 | 66 | 69 |
| 6 weeks | 24 | 41 | 38 | 39 | 42 | 42 |
| 4 months | 13 | 26 | 26 | 25 | 27 | 28 |

(Martin 1978; Martin and Monk 1982; Martin and White 1988; White et al. 1992; Foster et al. 1997; Hamlyn et al. 2002).

In 1999, the government specifically shifted its focus to one of targeting breastfeeding as a means to reducing inequalities in health (DoH 1999), related to the striking demographic variations in breastfeeding rates (Hamlyn *et al.* 2002). For example, 78 per cent of mothers aged thirty or above commenced breastfeeding compared to 46 per cent of mothers aged less than twenty. The incidence of breastfeeding in London and the south-east was 81 per cent compared to 61 per cent in the north of England. These variations correlated with socio-economic differences and, although there were increases in the number of women in socially excluded areas commencing breastfeeding, there were still striking differentials. In the UK, 85 per cent of mothers classified to higher occupations breastfed initially, compared with 73 per cent of mothers in intermediate occupations, 59 per cent in lower occupations and 52 per cent among those mothers who had never worked (Hamlyn *et al.* 2002).

The government (DoH 1999) therefore highlighted that infant feeding practices were an issue related to inequity. This public health issue was underlined in the government's NHS Plan, in which a commitment to increase breastfeeding rates by 2004 formed part of the proposed strategy to improve diet and nutrition (DoH 2000). The NHS Plan prioritised the reduction of health inequalities, and highlighted that lower levels of breastfeeding contributed to increased morbidity in lower socio-economic groups, with particular reference to cancers and coronary health. The Maternity Care Working Party (2001) document *Modernising Maternity Care: A Commissioning Toolkit for Primary Care Trusts in England*, in line with the government position, advocated that service-providers should demonstrate effective breastfeeding policies and practices that ensured ongoing support to breastfeeding mothers. Further commitment to increasing breastfeeding rates was reflected in *Improvement, Expansion and Reform: The Next Three Years' Priorities and Planning Framework, 2003–2006* (DoH 2002). This required all NHS Primary Care Trusts to facilitate an audited increase in their breastfeeding initiation rates by two per centage points per year with particular focus on women from disadvantaged groups. The momentum for promotion of breastfeeding continues with the recent publication of two further public health documents *Choosing Health* (DoH 2005a) and *Choosing a Better Diet* (DoH 2005b). Again, these documents emphasise the connections between socio-economic deprivation and sub-optimal diet and infant feeding practices.

### Breastfeeding support organisations in the UK

A concern for the loss of community-based, woman-centred, embodied and experiential knowledge related to breastfeeding led to the development of a range of breastfeeding support organisations, some international, others national. The La Leche League (LLL) was founded in 1956 in the US in response to the breastfeeding rates having dropped to just over 20 per cent (LLL 2003a). This organisation became established in the UK in the 1970s. The LLL ten-point philosophy (LLL 2003b) and statement of purpose (LLL 2003c) is explicit in associating long-term breastfeeding with good mothering and its organisational approach reflects this overtly essentialist position (Bobel 2001). The predominant support infrastructure of the LLL is through the development of peer support networks within local communities, specifically those in which women are least likely to breastfeed (LLL 2003d). The peer supporters are mothers who have breastfed or are still breastfeeding. They are provided with a short programme of training that involves understanding their personal experiences and being able to provide mother-to-mother support.

The National Childbirth Trust was established in the UK in 1956 with a focus upon re-establishing birth and breastfeeding as natural and empowering experiences for women (Carter 1995). The Association for Breastfeeding Mothers was founded in 1980 (ABM 2003). The fourth voluntary organisation to become established in the UK was the Breastfeeding Network (BfN 2003). This was founded in 1997 by a group of breastfeeding counsellors from the NCT, who objected to the organisation considering sponsorship from a group of chain stores that produced its own brand of infant formula. The BfN has a constitution that now ensures independence from commercial influence and it has a specific interest in providing 'outreach' breastfeeding support centres within socially deprived communities.

Despite philosophical differences between these support groups, their fundamental approach is woman-centred and non-directive. The NCT, ABM and BfN provide support to breastfeeding mothers through support groups and one-to-one supporter-to-mother contact, by telephone or home visit. The comprehensive programme of education has a strong reflexive component allowing the trainees to debrief on their own experiences. The trainees are supported in gaining person-centred counselling skills which include empathic understanding, unconditional positive regard (non-judgemental acceptance) and genuineness (Rogers 1961). Central to this approach is active listening and validating women in making their own decisions. In this way, supporters combine a collective knowledge of the principles of effective breastfeeding with an individualised woman-to-woman approach that acknowledges women's experiential and embodied knowledge and their own unique circumstances.

## International initiatives

Concerns within individual countries reflected a larger global effort to increase breastfeeding initiation and continuation rates by attempting initially to reverse the marketing of infant feeding, and later the entrenched medical routines, affecting infant feeding practices. This stemmed from growing international public concern during the 1970s in relation to the aggressive and unscrupulous marketing techniques used by multinational infant formula companies and their deleterious effects across the globe. The public outrage was initiated by the *New Internationalist* magazine, which prompted War on Want to publish *The Baby Killer* (Muller 1974), describing the advertising activities of the key milk manufacturers. Other publications followed, such as *Commerciogenic Malnutrition,* by Jelliffe (1972). As a result of the controversy, the World Health Organisation (WHO) and United Nations Children's Fund (UNICEF) convened a meeting in 1979 on Infant and Young Child Feeding. This meeting resulted in a commitment to form an *International Code of Marketing of Breast-Milk Substitutes* (WHO 1981). The WHO Code, as it is commonly abbreviated to, was established in 1981 in order to protect and encourage breastfeeding and to control inappropriate marketing practices used to sell products for artificial feeding (International Baby Food Action Network 1993). The WHO Code has now been internationally endorsed but success in implementation is dependent on government commitment, public awareness, strength of powerful vested interests and the dominance of western techno-medicine. Governments that embrace capitalism as their mode of production are reluctant to alienate the multinational companies, as they possess considerable political and economic power. In such societies profit and capital accumulation come first, with inevitable conflict in relation to a national health agenda.

In 1989, following sporadic international implementation of the WHO Code and continuing decline in breastfeeding in many countries, a renewed effort was made to reverse the global trend towards the use of infant formula and raise the momentum of political pressure on the infant formula companies. WHO and UNICEF published a joint statement *Protecting, Promoting and Supporting Breastfeeding* (WHO/UNICEF 1989). This statement included 'Ten Steps To Successful Breastfeeding', hereafter abbreviated to the Ten Steps (listed below). The Ten Steps were constructed by WHO/UNICEF to reflect what the two organisations felt were the crucial principles emerging from relevant research. This research underpinning the Ten Steps is summarised in a related document (WHO 1998). However, many health-care facilities were already involved in implementing some or all of these practices within maternity services to varying degrees. In 1990, WHO issued *The Innocenti Declaration on the Protection, Promotion and Support of Breastfeeding* (WHO/UNICEF 1990). This internationally endorsed declaration contained a comprehensive set of social policy targets to be reached by governments to assist a change of culture and facilitate increased breastfeeding initiation and duration rates. The declaration also contained a commitment to ensure that all maternity facilities meet the Ten Steps. At the 1990 World Summit for Children, the Convention on the Rights of the Child was ratified and the represented governments reiterated their commitment to the Ten Steps and to banning distribution of free and low-cost breast-milk substitutes to maternity facilities (Grant 1995).

### Ten Steps to Successful Breastfeeding

Every facility providing maternity services and care for newborn infants should:

1 Have a written breastfeeding policy that is routinely communicated to all healthcare staff.
2 Train all healthcare staff in skills necessary to implement the breastfeeding policy.

3   Inform all pregnant women about the benefits and management of breastfeeding.
4   Help mothers initiate breastfeeding within half an hour of birth.
5   Show mothers how to breastfeed and how to maintain lactation even if they are separated from their infants.
6   Give newborn infants no food or drink other than breast milk, unless medically indicated.
7   Practise rooming-in, allowing mothers and infants to remain together 24 hours a day.
8   Encourage breastfeeding on demand.
9   Give no artificial teats or pacifiers (also called dummies or soothers) to breastfeeding infants.
10   Foster the establishment of breastfeeding support groups and refer mothers to them on discharge from the hospital or clinic.

(WHO/UNICEF 1989: iv)

In 1991 WHO/UNICEF launched its global 'Baby Friendly Hospital Initiative' (BFHI). The purpose of this initiative was to support the development of an infrastructure by maternity care facilities which enabled them to implement the Ten Steps (WHO/UNICEF 1989). WHO and UNICEF were then involved in setting up national teams in participating countries, with the remit of co-ordinating and monitoring implementation in hospitals. Baby Friendly accreditation is issued to those deemed to have reached a minimum externally auditable standard in relation to the Ten Steps.

The comprehensive BFHI initiative aims to remove or reduce many of the hospital-based constraints that disadvantage breastfeeding women. Examples include the banning of advertising of breast-milk substitutes in maternity hospitals and removal of hospital nurseries. The mode of implementation of the BFHI has involved what Wright (1998) describes, in relation to the general politicisation of culture, as a deliberate unsettling and replacing of a dominant ideology that stems from medical dogma that has evolved over the past century. This requires not just political activity but the making of interventions in 'culture', involving manipulation of words and renaming and redefining key concepts. It could therefore be argued that one aim is to create a new ideology which, as Wright describes, 'becomes so naturalised, taken for granted and "true" that alternatives are beyond the limits of the thinkable' (5).

This global solution is appealing when one takes into account the devastation that the introduction of western medical dogma and commercial activity has had upon non-western communities and women's birthing and breastfeeding experiences. Women in some countries are labouring and birthing on uncovered metal trolleys, in lithotomy position, with their babies being extracted, removed and separated to a stark nursery and fed breast-milk substitutes (Lang, personal communication). The effects of poverty and lack of access to clean water upon the lives of babies and families when women utilise breast-milk substitutes for their babies are equally devastating (Dykes 1997).

The need for reversal of such inhumane practices is urgent and pressing and implementation of the BFHI has been associated with significant increases in breastfeeding initiation and duration rates (Prasad and Costello 1995; Cattaneo and Buzzetti 2001; Kramer *et al.* 2001; Philipp *et al.* 2001, 2003). However, the initiative is challenging to implement in that it advocates the making of relatively uniform changes across the globe in enormously diverse cultural settings. Even within one country, the mechanism by which change is managed and sustained will inevitably be influenced by the organisational culture of the maternity hospital within which the initiative is implemented. To add to the complexity a maternity hospital may be at various levels of engagement with the BFHI.

The certificate of commitment is awarded to hospitals that are intending to apply to be assessed for Baby Friendly accreditation in the future and have made specific preliminary progress towards that goal. Some hospitals are implementing aspects of the research underpinning the Ten Steps without any specific reference to the BFHI. This may or may not involve use of some of the BFHI resources such as leaflets and posters. Other hospitals have received Baby Friendly accreditation and are engaged in maintaining the standards required pending reassessment. Some hospitals have lost Baby Friendly accreditation due to a failed reassessment but are working towards reapplication. Other hospitals have lost the award and have decided to stop engaging with the initiative, although they may still retain a substantial connection with the principles underpinning the Ten Steps. This means that women using maternity services may believe that the hospital is Baby Friendly even when the hospital is not accredited, and this can damage the reputation of the initiative.

The most recent international initiative to be launched and potentially the most significant is the *Global Strategy for Infant and Young Child Feeding* (WHO 2003). This strategy was developed through a highly participatory global consultation process lasting two years. It is grounded on epidemiological and scientific evidence, while recognising the complex political and socio-cultural influences upon infant feeding practices.

The strategy's aim is to 'improve – through optimal feeding – the nutritional status, growth and development, health, and thus the survival of infants and young children' (6). Central to the strategy is the recommendation that infants are exclusively breastfed for the first six months of life and thereafter receive nutritionally adequate and safe complementary foods, with breastfeeding continuing for up to two years of age or beyond. It recognises that there are situations in which there may be exceptionally difficult circumstances for women, for example if they are HIV-positive and it elaborates upon ways of supporting women in these specific situations.

It is envisaged that the strategy will act as a catalyst for revitalising international attention towards the impact of feeding practices on the well-being of infants and young children. To achieve optimal infant and young child feeding practices the strategy calls for a renewed commitment to the WHO *International Code of Marketing of Breast-Milk Substitutes* (WHO 1981), the *Innocenti*

*Declaration on the Protection, Promotion and Support of Breastfeeding* (WHO 1990) and the Baby Friendly Hospital Initiative (WHO/UNICEF 1989). The strategy places particular emphasis upon the importance of community-based networks offering mother-to-mother support, and the need for trained breastfeeding counsellors to work closely with and/or within the healthcare system. This emphasis is based on the growing evidence that mother-to-mother support schemes and effective role-modelling are key to the restoration of breastfeeding as a cultural norm within communities around the world in which breastfeeding has progressively become a marginal activity (Dykes 2003, 2005c).

The strategy calls upon governments to develop, implement and evaluate a comprehensive national policy on infant and young child feeding and thereby to enable full operationalisation of its aims. This requires social, political and economic changes and concomitant public investment to be made to remove the constraints upon women in achieving and maintaining optimum infant and young child feeding practices. The extent to which the strategy is implemented across the globe will, as with the WHO Code, relate to government commitment, prioritisation and competing political agendas.

## Contemporary challenges

Despite the international, national and local initiatives that aim to protect, promote and support optimal infant feeding practices in industrialised communities, breastfeeding remains a challenge for many women. A growing body of qualitative research highlights the reasons why women do not breastfeed at all, prefer to partially breastfeed or discontinue breastfeeding early. This relates to a range of dilemmas and paradoxes surrounding breastfeeding. First, while the general view that 'breast is best' has become ideologically pervasive there are multiple constraints upon women in maintaining breastfeeding. There is growing pressure upon women to be a part of the paid workforce and this is paralleled by the growing emphasis upon the importance of breastfeeding, and increasingly exclusive breastfeeding, for six months (WHO 2003; Kramer and Kakuma 2003). Blum (1999) refers to these two contradictory trends in the US: the dramatic increase in mothers' wage-earning activities and the revival of breastfeeding prescriptions. She asserts that 'these two trends "work" through (and on) maternal bodies – bodies which have to get out into the public sphere, to seek autonomy, but also to engage in a most interdependent, private and time consuming act' (42).

In addition to this double imperative to 'work' and breastfeed, many women in the UK still feel dissonant about breastfeeding in public. This relates to the inherent ambiguities between breastfeeding as a maternal activity and breasts being increasingly and ever more explicitly displayed throughout every media channel as sexual items (Hawkins and Heard 2001; Pain *et al.* 2001; Mahon-Daly and Andrews 2002). Breastfeeding is still portrayed in the media and experienced by many women, particularly in socially deprived communities, as a marginal and liminal activity, rarely seen and barely spoken about (Hoddinott and Pill 1999a,

1999b, Henderson *et al.* 2000; Mahon-Daly and Andrews 2002). Women therefore continue to constantly negotiate the places and spaces in which they breastfeed (Pain *et al.* 2001; Mahon-Daly and Andrews 2002). Qualitative research also highlights that women continue to lack confidence in their ability to breastfeed (Hoddinott and Pill 1999a, 1999b; Blyth *et al.* 2002) and in particular their capacity to provide sufficient milk for their babies (Dykes and Williams 1999; Hawkins and Heard 2001; Dykes 2002, 2005a; Hamlyn *et al.* 2002).

This emerging body of qualitative research points to the need for understanding women's decisions related to infant feeding, through a socio-cultural conceptual lens. In addition to these socio-cultural constraints, women repeatedly report that the support from health professionals, particularly in hospital, is inadequate. The general failure to meet women's needs on postnatal wards in many industrialised countries has been repeatedly highlighted (Filshie *et al.* 1981; Stamp and Crowther 1994; Bondas-Salonen 1998; Garcia *et al.* 1998; Yelland *et al.* 1998; Rice *et al.* 1999; Singh and Newburn 2000; Briscoe *et al.* 2002).

Breastfeeding women are carrying out a partially learned activity which, in the absence of exposure during the socialisation process, combined with low levels of knowledge and support within a given community, requires support from health professionals. This is particularly the case when a women enters a postnatal ward where she is often separated from her family and friends for long periods throughout the day and night. In the UK, for example, the steepest decline in breastfeeding rates occurs during the first week, with 16 per cent of women who commenced breastfeeding in 2000 having stopped altogether by one week (Hamlyn *et al.* 2002). This is the period during which women spend time in hospital. The three key reasons given by UK women for discontinuing breastfeeding in hospital were: the baby fussing and/or not latching onto his/her mother's breast; sore or cracked nipples; and the mother's perception that she has insufficient milk to satisfy her baby (Foster *et al.* 1997; Hamlyn *et al.* 2002).

A number of international studies have focused specifically on the influence of the timing of postnatal discharge upon women's breastfeeding patterns in the UK (Winterburn and Fraser 2000), Sweden (Waldenstrom *et al.* 1987; Svedulf *et al.* 1998) and North America (Margolis and Schwartz 2000; Sheehan *et al.* 2001; McKeever *et al.* 2002). However, the results are equivocal due to heterogeneity of the studies and methodological limitations. McKeever *et al.* (2002) randomised women into two groups, a standard care and length of hospital stay versus earlier postnatal discharge with additional support from nurses who were also lactation consultants. The latter group were significantly more likely to sustain breastfeeding. However, as with other studies (Margolis and Schwartz 2000), this is more a comparison of types of support rather than 'place', in that in the early discharge group, women were receiving additional support from a health professional with a specific interest in breastfeeding. This support tends to increase breastfeeding duration (de Oliveira *et al.* 2001; Sikorski *et al.* 2004). Winterburn and Fraser (2000) randomised women into early (6–48 hours) or longer (3–7 days) postnatal discharges and reported no significant differences in breastfeeding rates.

However, they acknowledge that a serious problem with the study stemmed from women's reluctance to remain in hospital, an important finding in itself! Indeed, Sheehan *et al.*'s (2001) survey leads to the conclusion that a postpartum stay of over 48 hours constitutes a 'risk factor' for early discontinuation of breastfeeding (218). In summary, remaining in hospital versus early postnatal discharge does not appear to be of benefit to breastfeeding women and, as Brown *et al.* (2003) confirm, has no significant impact upon breastfeeding rates.

International studies have been conducted evaluating supportive interventions in hospital, usually in the form of breastfeeding information packages issued to women by individuals with specialist skills (Grossman *et al.* 1990; Redman *et al.* 1995; Hoyer and Horvat 2000; Porteous *et al.* 2000). However, the packages of information tend to be pre-defined by the researchers, and as most interventions involve an element of community follow-through, the isolated effect of the hospital support is difficult to evaluate. A systematic evaluation by Sikorski *et al.* (2004) demonstrated that such interventions increase the numbers of women breastfeeding their babies until the age of two months. However, they exercise caution in interpreting the research, as the supportive interventions during the postnatal period, levels of expertise of supporters and adherence to the support protocols were diverse and poorly defined.

Research has also been conducted to evaluate very focused interventions to improve women's skills at attaching their baby to their breast. However, the results of such prescriptive studies to date are varied; for example Righard and Alade (1992) demonstrated a statistically significant increase in continuation rates in Scandinavia. Subsequent studies have not produced statistically significant improvements (Schy *et al.* 1996; Henderson *et al.* 2001; Woods *et al.* 2002). However, Schy *et al.* (1996) highlighted as a result of a factor analysis associated with their study that professional encouragement, satisfaction with the experience and familial relationships were important to women. This finding suggests that more research is needed related to women's experiences of breastfeeding in hospital to elicit factors which *they* perceive to be important in relation to early breastfeeding.

A synthesis of the literature that focuses on the influence of professional encounters upon women's perception of their early breastfeeding experiences illustrates the ways in which women need support with breastfeeding. The reverse of these categories make women feel unsupported; for example encouragement contrasts with discouragement.

Women repeatedly state that emotional support is crucial, including a sense of being cared for and the staff showing concern and empathy (Tarkka and Paunonen 1996; Bondas-Salonen 1998; Bowes and Domokos 1998; Svedulf *et al.* 1998; Tarkka *et al.* 1998; Vogel and Mitchell 1998; Whelan and Lupton 1998; Hoddinott and Pill 2000; Hauck *et al.* 2002). The forming of a relationship with the health carer(s) is valued although not necessarily expected (Vogel and Mitchell 1998; Whelan and Lupton 1998; Hoddinott and Pill 2000; Porteous *et al.* 2000; Raisler 2000; Hauck *et al.* 2002; McKeever *et al.* 2002). Help with coping with emotions (Hoddinott and Pill 2000), general professional sensitivity (Mozingo *et al.* 2000) and protection from embarrassment caused by learning to breastfeed in front of others, or feeling that it is offensive to others (Vogel and Mitchell 1998, Hoddinott and Pill 2000, Hauck 2002), all relate to feeling cared for. Women welcome receiving adequate staff time and availability in contrast to feeling rushed (Tarkka and Paunonen 1996; Bondas-Salonen 1998; Bowes and Domokos 1998; Svedulf 1998; Tarkka *et al.* 1998; Vogel and Mitchell 1998; Whelan and Lupton 1998; Hoddinott and Pill 2000; Hauck *et al.* 2002; Hong *et al.* 2003). They prefer a quiet hospital environment in which the mother is assisted in feeling rested, confident and less anxious (Ball 1994; Tarkka and Paunonen 1996; Bondas-Salonen 1998; Tarkka *et al.* 1998; Vogel and Mitchell 1998).

Professional encouragement and confidence-building are highly valued by women (Ball 1994; Schy *et al.* 1996; Humenick *et al.* 1998; Svedulf *et al.* 1998; Hoddinott and Pill 2000; Gill 2001; McCreath *et al.* 2001; Hauck *et al.* 2002; Ingram *et al.* 2002). This includes reassurance of the baby's well-being (Hoddinott and Pill 2000) and that early difficulties may be overcome (Mozingo *et al.* 2000; Hauck 2002).

In relation to the provision of information, women value respect for individuality versus standardised advice (Hauck *et al.* 2002; Hoddinott and Pill 2000) and provision of information that is realistic, useful and accurate (Rajan 1993; Svedulf *et al.* 1998; Whelan and Lupton 1998; Hoddinott and Pill 2000; Mozingo *et al.* 2000; Gill 2001; Hauck *et al.* 2002; McKeever *et al.* 2002; McLeod 2002; Hong *et al.* 2003). This information needs to be given by staff who are knowledgeable about breastfeeding and able to teach the necessary skills (Bowes and Domokos 1998; Vogel and Mitchell 1998; Raisler 2000; Ingram *et al.* 2002; McKeever *et al.* 2002). The information also needs to be consistent (Rajan 1993; Ball 1994; Tarkka and Paunonen 1996; Vogel and Mitchell 1998; Hoddinott and Pill 2000; Mozingo *et al.* 2000; Simmons 2002a, 2002b; Hauck *et al.* 2002; Ingram *et al.* 2002). In one study, women explicitly referred to the need to be respected for their own knowledge, rather than feeling that expert knowledge was unchallengeable (Bowes and Domokos 1998). This relates to women's desire for facilitation of their own knowledge and problem-solving abilities, rather than simply being advised as to what to do (Whelan and Lupton 1998; Hoddinott and Pill 2000; Gill 2001).

Women generally welcome practical assistance with breastfeeding when required (Rajan 1993; Hoddinott and Pill 2000; Mozingo *et al.* 2000; Raisler 2000; Hong *et al.* 2003). This, however, needs to be combined with sensitive respect for body boundaries (Vogel and Mitchell 1998; Whelan and Lupton 1998; Hoddinott and Pill 2000; Mozingo *et al.* 2000; Ingram *et al.* 2002). Finally, assistance with maintaining existing networks of significant others, and the activation and establishment of supportive networks within the new situation, are important to women (Bondas-Salonen 1998; Tarkka *et al.* 1998).

These studies highlight the importance of women's satisfaction with the hospital experience while embarking on their breastfeeding project. Emotional support from staff with knowledge, time and supportive skills such as encouragement and sensitivity emerge as significant in relation to maternity service provision at this crucial time. However, this literature referred to has a number of key limitations. First, it takes little account of the culture in which women are supported (or are not supported) and second, it relates to what women say, which is crucial, but it does not involve observational data to supplement stories heard and told. Before moving on to refer to studies that have observed as well as heard about the experiences of breastfeeding women, I briefly refer to the cultural context within which many women commence breastfeeding.

## *'Seeing' the cultural context*

There is now a growing body of international research that relates to the influence of the culture/environment upon healthcare workers' abilities to 'care' (Davis-Floyd 1992; Street 1992; Davis-Floyd and St John 1998; Kirkham 1999; Woodward 2000; Stevens and McCourt 2001a; Kirkham and Stapleton 2001b; Lugina *et al.* 2001, 2002; Hughes *et al.* 2002; Ball *et al.* 2002; Hunter 2002, 2004, 2005; Deery 2003, 2005; Varcoe *et al.* 2003). The culture in which women learn to breastfeed and midwives provide (or do not provide) support is crucial to any critical study of the subject. It plays a key role in how women cope with their emotions, change of role and learning the new skills associated with motherhood. It is also crucial in its influence upon midwives and how they cope with *their* emotions and role. As McCourt and Percival (2000) state: 'the supportive or caring qualities of midwives cannot be readily separated from the organization of their work' (264).

Research in western industrialised countries, such as the UK and US, highlights the techno-medical, hierarchical, oppressive, gendered and separatist nature of the healthcare system in which health professionals are expected to work (Davis-Floyd 1992; Street 1992; Davis-Floyd and St. John 1998; Kirkham 1999; Kirkham and Stapleton 2001b and Ball *et al.* 2002). Kirkham focused upon the culture of National Health Service (NHS) midwifery in the UK in two major studies (Kirkham 1999; Ball *et al.* 2002). She refers to the hospital system, with its hierarchical and gendered agenda, as separating 'birth from life' and 'women from their wider social environment' (Kirkham 1999: 733). Within these institutions, Kirkham argues, skills of 'support, caring and being with women' become 'invisible' and very difficult for midwives to achieve (ibid.). Indeed, she describes some of the characteristics of life for UK midwives as akin to the conditions described by Freire (1972), in his *Pedagogy of the Oppressed* (Kirkham 1999). She also refers to the absence of a support infrastructure for the midwives who needed support in order to provide support for others (Kirkham 1999; Kirkham and Stapleton 2000; Ball *et al.* 2002).

Davis-Floyd and St John (1998) in the US provide further insight into the dehumanising effects of the hospital culture upon health professionals themselves, in a comprehensive qualitative study involving in-depth interviews with forty medical practitioners who had undergone a transformative journey to become healers. The practitioners described the 'separatist world view' inherent in the conventional healthcare system. They referred to the ways in which they had turned their own bodies into tools and abused that tool 'to make it continue to function in spite of overwork and high stress' (22). They had cut themselves off from their emotions leading to a sense of detachment and alienation. Davis-Floyd and St John (1998) highlight some of the effects of the hierarchy to include privileging of specialists and specialist knowledge and the subordination of the individual to the institution.

It seems, then, that any account of women's experiences of breastfeeding within hospital should not and cannot 'skirt around' the context within which their supporters are working and yet this is rarely addressed. A crucial way to focus specifically upon the hospital experience prospectively, and to 'see' as well as 'hear' what is happening, is to conduct a study that includes observation. However, there is a striking absence of ethnographic work conducted on postnatal wards and considerably less that focuses upon aspects of breastfeeding within the postnatal ward setting. Observational studies that focus upon breastfeeding women in postnatal wards include: practice development projects (Renfrew 1989); exploration of specific activities, for example supplementation with infant formula (Cloherty *et al.* 2004) or pacifier use (Victora *et al.* 1997); decision-making by women (Marchand and Morrow 1994) and general support for breastfeeding women (Gill 2001). However, these studies do not adopt a critical theory perspective nor do they specifically explore the organisational culture. In the remainder of this book I describe an in-depth critical ethnographic study exploring influences upon women's experiences of breastfeeding on UK postnatal wards. I commence, in Chapter 3, with a description of the ethnographic research and the underlying critical theoretical perspective that informed the study.

# Chapter 3

# Participating in production

## Introduction

In this chapter I discuss the critical theory perspective underpinning this book, the conduct of the ethnography, and I describe the hospital culture within which women commence their breastfeeding journey. I illustrate the hospital culture with some of my ethnographic observations and narratives of breastfeeding women and of midwives. This provides the context for the ensuing chapters in that I emphasise not only the medical nature of the experience for mothers but the 'factory-like' working conditions for midwives.

## A critical medical anthropological perspective

The central focus of this study is upon culture and the ways in which human experiences and interactions are influenced, negotiated and understood. Culture and enculturation are crucial factors in determining and influencing the way we see the world. These concepts are defined by Helman:

> Culture is a set of guidelines (both explicit and implicit) which individuals inherit as particular members of a society, and which tells them how to *view* the world, how to experience it emotionally, and how to *behave* in it in relation to other people, to supernatural forces or gods, and to the natural environment. It also provides them with a way of transmitting these guidelines to the next generation – by the use of symbols, language, art and ritual. To some extent, culture can be seen as an inherited 'lens' through which the individual perceives and understands the world that he inhabits, and learns how to live within it. Growing up within any society is a form of *enculturation*, whereby the individual slowly aquires the cultural lens of that society. Without such a shared perception of the world, both the cohesion and continuity of any human group would be impossible.
>
> (Helman 1994: 2–3)

Spradley (1980) defines culture as 'the acquired knowledge people use to interpret experience and generate behaviour' (6). Crucially, I agree with Spradley in avoiding cultural determinism, that is not seeing culture as simply programming individuals. As Spradley argues, culture should be viewed as a cognitive map acting as a reference and guide. It should not be seen as constraining the person to adopt only one course of action. Nevertheless, Spradley does acknowledge that culture does create in the person a taken-for-granted view of reality and in this sense individuals are somewhat culture-bound. In this way humans are able to exercise agency within their cultural parameters. This balance between enculturation and agency assists in understanding the differences between 'tacit knowledge', a knowledge that remains largely outside our immediate awareness, and 'explicit knowledge', a form of knowledge that people may communicate about with a relative ease (Spradley 1980: 7). I return to the notion of culture in subsequent sections, but first discuss my theoretical perspective.

A critical medical anthropological perspective underpinned this study. Critical medical anthropology constitutes a critical perspective upon traditional forms of medical anthropology that was concerned primarily with observing and describing health-related encounters and phenomena without challenge. The theoretical basis for critical medical anthropology stems from critical theory. Critical theory is commonly associated with the Frankfurt School of Critical Inquiry and especially the work of Habermas (1972), and political theorists to include Marx (1970), Gramsci (1971) and Freire (1972). The definition proposed by Kincheloe and McClaren of a researcher or theorist embracing critical theory is useful in illustrating the key tenets of this perspective:

> We are defining a criticalist as a researcher or theorist who attempts to use her or his work as a form of social or cultural criticism and who accepts certain basic assumptions: that all thought is fundamentally mediated by power relations that are socially and historically constituted; that facts can never be isolated from the domain of values or removed from some form of ideological inscription; that the relationship between concept and object and between signifier and signified is never stable or fixed and is often mediated by the social relations of capitalist production and consumption; that language is central to the form of subjectivity (conscious and unconscious awareness); that certain groups in any society are privileged over others [...] that oppression has many faces.
>
> (Kincheloe and McClaren 1994: 139–140)

Kincheloe and McClaren (1994) also include under their broad definition of critical theory some post-structuralist theories such as those of Foucault. This inclusivity needs careful clarification when considering perspectives on, for example, ideology and power; a discussion that I return to. In general, then, the critical perspective stands in contrast to interpretevist approaches in that it seeks to move beyond understanding, to capturing issues related to ideology, power, conflict and oppression. In this way it seeks to be transformative. Critical medical anthropology applies this critical perspective to the anthropological study of health. It has a particular focus upon blending the macro-perspective with the micro-perspective as a means of constructing an integrated paradigm (Singer 1990). A balance between macro and micro is at the heart of the critical medical anthropology perspective:

> It takes positions on the medicalisation of every day life in contemporary society, which it opposes; on biomedicine as a form of power, domination, and social control, which it also opposes; and on mind–body dualism, again in opposition. Its intellectual debts are to Marx, Gramsci, the Frankfurt school of critical theory, phenomenology and political economy. Its agenda includes critique of medicine as an institution, cultural criticism focused on the domain of health, analysis of capitalism in the macro-politics of health care systems and the micro-politics of bodies and persons, addition of historical depth to cultural analysis, and critique of allegedly non-critical medical anthropology.
>
> (Csordas 1988: 417)

## Macro-perspective

Central to the critical medical anthopology perspective are power structures, ideology, hegemony and oppression (Gramsci 1971; Freire 1972; Kapferer 1988; Bellamy 1995). Emphasis is placed upon:

> Particular sets of meanings, because they have come into being in and out of the give-and-take of social existence [and] exist to serve hegemonic interests. Each set of meanings supports particular power structures, resists moves towards greater equity, and harbours oppression, manipulation and other modes of injustice and unfreedom.
>
> (Crotty 1998: 59–60)

Hegemony as a concept was a major political contribution developed by Gramsci (1971). Gramsci was an Italian neo-Marxist. He wrote about hegemony in his prison diaries whilst in a fascist prison, where he died. His diaries were later translated by Hoare and Nowell Smith in 1971. Gramsci emphasised 'the ideological ascendancy of one or more groups or classes over others in civil society' (Bellamy 1995: 33) and the transmission of economic power through ideology and culture. The Gramscian concept of hegemony presents culture as dynamic and central in the study of social processes, historical in nature and deeply embedded in human beings and existence (Kapferer 1988). Ideology refers to a shared set of fundamental beliefs about the world that justify 'what is' (Thomas 1993: 8) and these ideas serve as 'weapons for social interests' (Berger and Luckmann 1966: 18).

The political economy of health perspective has had a particular influence upon the development of critical medical anthropology. Its focus is upon the relationships between capitalist modes of production, medical practice, health and illness (Gough 1979; Frankenburg 1980; Doyal and Pennell 1979; Navarro 1992; Gray 1993; Illich 1995). Doyal and Pennell (1979), for example, illustrate the contradictions between the goals of improving health and the imperatives of capital accumulation inherent within the capitalist mode of production. They also highlight the ways in which particular forms of medical practice have developed within societies that embrace the capitalist mode of production. They argue that medical techniques and technology are the 'product of a particular conjunction of social, economic and political forces' (292). Therefore, the existence of any particular medical practice and its associated technology should be understood in relation to the activities of powerful groups within society whose interests are furthered by the development, maintenance and proliferation of such technologies.

Western biomedicine may be seen as iatrogenic in nature, that is, potentially or actually harmful (Illich 1995). Despite rhetoric about equal access to healthcare through national services, the social organisation of medicine within nations employing the capitalist mode of production still reinforces socio-economic, sexual and racial divisions (Doyal and Pennell 1979; Navarro 1992; Gray 1993; Illich 1995). Western capitalist modes of production have both contributed towards and failed to alleviate the burden of disease still experienced by huge sections of the population in underdeveloped parts of the world (Doyal and Pennell 1979; Gray 1993; George 1994). Finding solutions to these problems is highly challenging and complex and having a socialist government would not necessarily provide a better alternative, unless it addressed the following:

> A socialist health service would not only have to provide equal access to medical care but would also have to address itself seriously to such problems as how to demystify medical knowledge and how to break down barriers of authority and status among health workers themselves and also between workers and consumers. Indeed, the whole notion of 'treating patients' – of seeing them as passive recipients of medical expertise – would need to be rethought.
>
> (Doyal and Pennell 1979: 194)

### Micro-perspective

The micro-perspective enables a:

> close-up view of local populations and their lifeways, systems of meaning, motivations for action, points of view, and daily experiences and emotions. It is concerned with how the system works – to include how players act and feel and know, where the contradictions and arenas of social conflict lie, and how power is distributed and exercised.
>
> (Singer 1990: 297)

The micro-focus upon a cultural milieu could relate to a specific community, group of people or organisation such as a hospital. This culture, or an aspect of it, is observed and described in detail.

The micro-perspective then probes further into the lived experiences of individuals within that situation or context. With regard to health research, notions of embodiment and embodied experience are central. It is only in the past two to three decades that 'bodies' have 'come back' within the social sciences in recognition that 'the corporeal grounds the existential' and 'whatever is done to bodies is political' (Frank 1990: 132). The body used to be bypassed by the macro-sociological view that emphasised the political economic processes involved in social control, and the micro-sociological perspective that focused upon social influences on behaviour but not embodied experience (Lupton 1994). Critical medical anthropology, however, restored this balance with embodied experiences becoming a key focus (Frankenberg 1980; Csordas 1988, 1994a, 1994b; Singer 1990; Lyon and Barbalet 1994).

The embodied experience is an area that cannot be ignored in any health-related study. As Merleau-Ponty (1962) notes, 'my body is the pivot of the world' and 'I am conscious of my body via the world' (82). Kapferer (1988) likewise highlights that it is within the body that life is experienced and organised. He argues that in traditional medical anthropology there has been a development of abstract categories and their relationships without emphasis upon embodiment. The body was commonly regarded as an expressive vehicle of a world that surrounds the body, 'the mind is separated from the body, the mental from the material, and the historical, social and political from their embodied realisation' (426). This traditional anthropological view saw the body as simply inscribed by culture.

Within critical medical anthropology there is now increasing resistance to the original classifications of the body in classic terms, that is: perception, or use of the senses; practice or techniques of the body; parts or anatomy; bodily processes; and body products or secretions (Csordas 1994b). Rather than this representational perspective there is growing engagement with experiences stemming from the body and the associated lived experiences of being in the world (Kapferer 1988; Csordas 1994b; Lyon and Barbalet 1994). This perspective draws upon phenomenology (Merleau-Ponty 1962). Critical medical anthropologists tend to see a person's body as an active agent in its own construction (Lyon and Barbalet 1994) thus balancing structure and agency in viewing people as active agents, while acknowledging that there are many socio-cultural constraints upon them.

### Transformative action

Central to the medical anthropological approach is transformative action. This relates to Freire's (1972) philosophy, as articulated by Peters and Lankshear (1994), that:

Human development is based upon a certain quality of awareness: awareness of our temporality, our 'situatedness' in history, and our reality as being capable of transformation through action in collaboration with others [...]. Progress from naive to critical consciousness involves conscientization. This is the process by which we learn to perceive social, political, and economic contradictions and become involved in the struggle to overcome them; to identify 'limit situations' for what they are and confront them with 'limit acts'. In this very process we enter history as subjects, humanizing ourselves, becoming more fully human.

(Peters and Lankshear 1994: 181)

Active resistance may be undertaken to challenge an ideology, public knowledge or authority that sets guidelines, policies or instructions (Street 1992). The most effective way in which to engage in active resistance is through collective action and challenge (Freire 1972; Street 1992). This powerful form of resistance, in turn, yields transformation and emancipatory change to a political agenda (Freire 1972; Singer 1990). This transformative action is possible through awareness-raising of the socio-political and economic 'limit situations' and a practical endeavour to counter these situations with 'limit acts' (Freire 1972). In this way, the macro–micro connections, so fundamental to critical medical anthropology, are maintained. To confront limit acts requires collective action and this in turn requires collective conscientisation (Freire 1972).

## A woman-centred perspective

As a central focus within this book relates to the empowerment of women, I necessarily engage with aspects of feminism. In essence, the feminist theoretical perspective centres upon the challenge to dominant assumptions, inequities and social injustice that relate to women. It is critical in the sense that it seeks transformation and emancipation. However, feminism covers a diverse range of theoretical perspectives that reflect the many contentious phases in its development. Tong (1998) illustrates the diversities within feminism by categorising key feminist perspectives taking into account the interconnections with other theoretical perspectives. She devotes a chapter of her book to each of the following: 'liberal feminism', 'radical feminism', 'Marxist and socialist feminism', 'psychoanalytical and gender feminism', 'existentialist feminism', 'postmodern feminism', 'multicultural and global feminism' and 'ecofeminism'. While many feminists avoid such demarcations, such labels do:

signal to the broader public that feminism is not a monolithic ideology, that all feminists do not think alike, and that, like all other time-honoured modes of thinking, feminist thought has a past as well as a present and future [...]. They help mark the range of different approaches, perspectives and frameworks a variety of feminists have used to shape both their explanations for women's oppression and their proposed solutions for its elimination.

(Tong 1998: 2)

In aligning myself with a political economy of health perspective, I am in agreement with those who see oppression of women as being strongly related to political, social and economic structures, with the capitalist mode of production being one such structure (Doyal and Pennel 1979; Martin 1987; Palmer 1993; Van Esterik 1994). I also recognise other forms of oppression of women stemming from the growth of a traditionally male-dominated medical system and sexual appropriation of women's bodies. I see capitalism and the techno-medical model of medicine as inextricably linked and contributing to a series of dualistic separations; mind–body, public–private, nature–culture, production– (re)production and maternal–sexual; all limiting possibilities for women (Doyal and Pennel 1979; Martin 1987; Van Esterik 1989a, 1989b,1994). I therefore see the need for transformative action to tackle financial inequities and the institutional and cultural practices that disempower women.

Breastfeeding is an embodied activity that women experience within a socio-cultural context. It has therefore posed enormous challenges for feminists, stemming from the well-rehearsed but little-resolved dualistic feminist debates related to sameness or difference. These debates focus upon women's dilemmas related to whether they would prefer to strive to be recognised and respected for their differences or sameness in relation to men (Humm 1992; Shildrick 1997). As Shildrick (1997) argues, on the one hand there is a celebration of femininity and difference bringing with it the risks of essentialism and locating women within a maternal role. On the other hand, there is celebration of sameness and equality with men. Consequently, feminists appear to find it very difficult to know where to locate themselves along the essentialist/non-essentialist continuum. This has led to a vacuum with regard to feminist critique related to breastfeeding that has only started to be addressed.

The feminist writings on breastfeeding appear to represent three key perspectives: historical (Apple 1987; Fildes 1986), a broadly political economy of health perspective (Van Esterik 1989a; 1994; Altergott 1991; Palmer 1993; Shelton 1994; Baumslag and Michels 1995; Galtry 2000) or a post-structuralist perspective (Maher 1992a; Carter 1995; Schmied 1998; Blum 1999; Schmied and Barclay 1999), although there are inevitably overlaps. I focus here upon the political-economic approaches and the post-structuralist perspective. The former tend to present breastfeeding as potentially transformative and empowering to women, but highlight the many socio-political and cultural constraints upon women. They highlight the interconnected impacts of medicalisation of breastfeeding, marketing of infant formula, and sexualisation of women's breasts upon women's choices, decisions and embodied experiences of breastfeeding (Van Esterik 1989a, 1989b; Altergott 1991; Palmer 1993; Shelton 1994; Baumslag and Michels 1995). Galtry adopts a very specific focus on the influence of labour relations and workplace legislation upon women's experiences of breastfeeding in the US (Galtry 1997a, 1997b, 1997c, 2000) and internationally (2003). The general emphasis for these authors is upon politically mediated reversal of constraints to enable and empower women across the globe to breastfeed. Van Esterik summarises this position:

> Breastfeeding is a feminist issue because it encourages women's self-reliance, confirms a woman's power to control her own body, challenges models of women as consumers and sex objects, requires a new interpretation of women's work, and encourages solidarity among women.
>
> (Van Esterik 1989b: 69)

The post-structuralist feminists argue that the position adopted by this politically motivated group of authors who they tend to label as 'breastfeeding advocates' are still fundamentally essentialist in their connection of women with their reproductive functions (Maher 1992a; Carter 1995; Blum 1999). Maher (1992a) presents this argument from a global anthropological perspective; Carter (1995) following interviews with working-class women who had their babies between 1920 and 1980 in the UK; Blum (1999) based on research with women in contemporary US; and Schmied following interviews with Australian women (Schmied 1998; Schmied and Barclay 1999). All critique what they see as a deterministic assumption that breastfeeding was, is or could be empowering for all women.

Engaging with the post-structuralist feminist literature required me to consider carefully my own position. To support me in this, in addition to turning to the post-structuralist writings of Foucault to which I return shortly, I also engaged with the writings of feminists who chart their journey from a less relativistic, standpoint position into post-structuralism and then locate themselves somewhere 'in between', drawing from both (Haraway 1991; Burman 1992; Stanley and Wise 1993; Hastrup 1995; Standing 1998; Pujol 1999; Willig 1999a, 1999b).

The critique of Burman (1992) is particularly illuminating in that she examines the need for a feminism that is neither positivistic nor totally relativistic, highlighting four areas where feminism and post-structuralism converge: they both pay attention to difference, that is, what dominant theories omit or repress; they make relative the practices of regulation, for example, medicine; they affirm reflexivity; and they highlight how practices of regulation do not exert their power without simultaneously producing resistance. In embracing aspects of post-structuralism, Burman (1992) warns that 'celebrating plurality and indeterminacy' may lead to 'total interpretative relativism' that disregards all models and theories (51). She thereby strongly argues for maintenance of the transformative and emancipatory potential of collective resistance embedded in the feminist project:

> Despite the focus on difference and dispersion, we need to retain the possibility of commitment to some unified theory to maintain the feminist project

of social transformation, and equally to ward off linguistic relativism by ensuring that the politics of the theory is not only theoretical [...]. We need to affirm for strategic purposes that there is some commonality in the positions and experiences of women by virtue of our subordination.

(Burman 1992: 48)

Standing (1998) likewise summarises some of these issues. As a feminist materialist she argues that post-structuralism was a:

vacuous theory, with no grounding in the material realities of everyday life. Power seemed to come from everywhere and nowhere. The emphasis on deconstruction seemed to me to alienate theory from practice, to individualize and leave me as a feminist, with nothing to organize around politically.

(Standing 1998: 196)

However, she reflects that her earlier views on power were rather simplistic and she proceeded to embrace some of the post-structuralist understandings regarding the diffuse nature of power and modes of resistance. This reflects my stance in relation to women and breastfeeding in that I primarily embrace a macro, political-economic perspective. However, partial engagement with post-structuralism provides me with a micro-perspective that reflects the complexity of women's experiences of breastfeeding. In this way I offer a synthesis that unites a macro-political perspective with a micro-perspective that stems from the meanings for women when engaging in a breastfeeding 'project' in a hospital setting.

## Post-structuralist perspectives on power

I now elaborate upon ways in which I engage with some of the post-structuralist thought of Foucault (1976, 1977, 1980, 1981), particularly in relation to surveillance. As stated, in the broad sense, Foucault's work is encompassed by the critical theory perspective (Kincheloe and McLaren 1994). However, while critical medical anthropology seeks to address the 'micro/macro nexus as a means of constructing an integrated paradigm', post-structuralism is more concerned with discourse, that is the 'social determinants of textual production' (Singer 1990: 297). While the two are not fundamentally incompatible, the pluralistic, relativist and non-interventionist stance encompassed by post-structuralism may lead to a de-politicised approach lacking in transformative potential. With this in mind, I draw upon Foucault's theory with caution but welcome its challenge for me to (re)look through a less deterministic lens at the issues. To clarify some of the convergences and divergences between these perspectives, I discuss aspects of power here, in that it is central to both critical medical anthropology and post-structuralism. However, there are fundamental differences as to its conceptualisation.

## Power and ideology

As stated, power structures, ideology, hegemony and oppression are central to the political economy of health perspective. Foucault's (1977, 1980) view of power differs in his opposition to the concept of dominant ideologies exerting an oppressive power. He does acknowledge the 'pyramidal organization' of power but he argues that this power is dispersed to the disciplinary apparatus (1977: 176). As Fairclough (1992) argues, Foucault's resistance to the concept of ideology and to the idea of analysis as a form of ideological critique arises from his relativism. A major distinguishing feature of Foucault's concept of power stems from his argument that power is not vertically transmitted down through the political-economic systems, with powerful groups of society simply oppressing and dominating those in less powerful positions. He sees power as diffuse, diverse, ambiguous and located everywhere in day-to-day relationships and encounters, with everyone being caught up in the mechanisms of power:

> Power is exercised rather than possessed; it is not the 'privilege', acquired or preserved, of the dominant class, but the overall effect of its strategic positions – an effect that is manifested and sometimes extended by the position of those who are dominated. Furthermore, this power is not exercised simply as an obligation or a prohibition on those 'who do not have it'; it invests them, is transmitted by them and through them; it exerts pressure upon them, just as they themselves, in their struggle against it, resist the grip it has on them.
>
> (Foucault 1977: 26–27)

Foucault is clear about what power is not:

> By power I do not mean 'Power' as a group of institutions and mechanisms that ensure the subservience of the citizens of a given state. By power I do not mean, either a mode of subjugation which in contrast to violence, has the form of the rule. Finally, I do not have in mind a general system of domination exerted by one group over another, a system whose effects, through successive derivations, pervade the entire social body.
>
> (Foucault 1981: 92)

Although Foucault (1977, 1980) makes reference to Panopticism as an architectural structure whereby power may be transmitted through the 'gaze', he emphasises the multidirectional nature of power within a surveillance system, arguing that power is everywhere, operating from top down, bottom up and laterally, with the supervisors being both objects and subjects of power:

> Power is everywhere; not because it embraces everything but because it comes from everywhere [...]. Power is not an institution, and not a structure; neither is it a certain strength we are endowed with; it is the name that one

attributes to a complex strategical situation in a particular society [...]. Power is not something that is acquired, seized, or shared, something that one holds on to or allows to slip away; power is exercised from innumerable points, in the interplay of non egalitarian and mobile relations.

(Foucault 1981: 93, 94)

Foucault (1980) refers to this dispersion of power as being ambiguous and passing through fine channels. It is a 'capillary' form of power that 'reaches into the very grain of individuals, touches their bodies and inserts itself into their actions and attitudes, their discourses, learning processes and everyday lives' (1980: 39). While, unlike Foucault, I see power as transmitted through ideology, I do, at least partially, embrace Foucault's notion of power as diffused through disciplinary surveillance (1977). This supports an understanding of the complex ways in which power is embedded and intertwined within cultural systems.

## Power and knowledge

Foucault links power and knowledge as inseparable, mutually dependent and reinforcing, arguing that, 'There is no power relation without the correlative constitution of a field of knowledge, nor any knowledge that does not presuppose and constitute at the same time power relations' (Foucault 1977: 27). To assist understanding of the ways in which the 'formation of knowledge and the increase of power regularly reinforce one another in a circular process' (224), Foucault takes us back to the eighteenth century, the era when the disciplines crossed the 'technological threshold'. Hospitals, for example, became:

Apparatuses such that any mechanism of objectification could be used in them as an instrument of subjection, and any growth of power could give rise in them to possible branches of knowledge; it was this link which made possible within the disciplinary element the formation of clinical medicine, child psychiatry, child psychology, educational psychology, the rationalization of labour. It is a double process, then: an epistemological 'thaw' through a refinement of power relations; a multiplication of the effects of power through the formation and accumulation of new forms of knowledge.

(Foucault 1977: 224)

In this way, Foucault points to the ability of the disciplines to 'define a certain field of empirical truth' (Gordan 1980: 237). However, he does not see knowledge as fundamentally oppressive, but as productive (Gordan 1980). Therefore, as Street (1992) argues, because Foucault views knowledge and power as inseparable, he must reject the notion of power as a medium through which emancipatory knowledge may be generated. This would imply a separation of power from knowledge, with 'knowledge being related to truth, and power being equated with oppression and repression' (101). He therefore sees a separation of the concepts of power and knowledge as repressive in that it enables power to hide its own mechanisms.

While I agree that power and knowledge are inextricably interconnected, I see powerful groups as maintaining their authoritative versions of knowing, to serve their ends, and in turn to oppress less dominant groups and their ways of knowing. In this way, I argue that challenging authoritative knowledges, their sources and modes of transmission has emancipatory potential (Freire 1972). However, engaging with Foucault's understanding of the mutual 'enwrapping, interaction and interdependence of power and knowledge' (Gordan 1980: 233) assists me in taking a 'middle' position that is neither wholly deterministic nor relativistic.

## Power and the body

One of the ways in which Foucault (1976, 1977, 1980, 1981) sees power as being transmitted is through the body and this constitutes a crucial focus within this book. Foucault (1976, 1977, 1981) conceptualises the body as a text inscribed upon, constructed and constituted by discourse. The notion of Panopticism, when transmitted to bodies, leads to an intense form of self-discipline and body management. While I agree with the potential for deep inscription of bodies by discourse, I disagree that the body may be viewed merely as a passive script to be inscribed by social structure. Like others, I argue that a person's body is also an agent in its own world construction (Fairclough 1992; Street 1992; Lyon and Barbalet 1994; Shildrik 1997). Again, in this way, I return to my position of balance between structure and agency, seeing women as active agents, while acknowledging that there are many socio-cultural constraints upon them.

While Foucault focused upon the body, he had little to say about women's bodies apart from commenting on their sexuality (1981) and yet, as Shildrik (1997) argues, the concept of the 'gaze' and its self-regulating potential is highly relevant to the female body. 'The imagery of nature unveiled before science, of the body stripped of its fleshy protection and penetrated by the empirical gaze is strongly gender-linked' (Shildrik 1997: 31). Foucault also neglected any reference to male dominance and women's bodies, but he did see the body and sexuality as 'central to the interplay of power and resistance', a crucial position within feminist perspectives (Shildrik 1997: 22).

While considerable insight may be drawn from Foucault's notion of the inscribed body, I argue that this must be balanced with a theory of embodiment. With regard to breastfeeding women, this synthesis is provided by Schmied (1998), who argues that maternal subjectivity and breastfeeding must be viewed as both an embodied experience and a discursive construction. I agree with Schmied (1998), and further assert that a third dimension, stemming from political economy of health, allows us to be ever aware of the profoundly political and medicalised nature of bodily experiences. Wherever there is discussion related to power and the body there must be reference to the various forms of resistance that I now refer to.

## Power and resistance

Foucault (1976, 1977, 1981) acknowledges resistance, but appears to see it as contained by power and posing no real threat. Bodies are depicted as docile, disciplined, obedient and accommodating. As Fairclough (1992) comments, 'the dominant impression is one of people being helplessly subjected to immovable systems of power' (57). Resistance is then 'spontaneous, individual and elusive' (Burman 1992: 50).

Whilst I agree that resistance may occur at an individual level, I argue that a balance is needed between the notions of structure and agency. I take a position along the continuum, seeing women not as docile scripts but as having some ability to actively negotiate their situations. However, I recognise that their projects in life such as mothering and feeding their babies are affected by multiple constraints that are discursive, cultural and political. Current arguments around passivity versus activity/agency appear to be somewhat polarised and tend to ignore the ways in which women may engage in both accommodation and resistance selectively, as they negotiate various expectations and constraints upon them (Street 1992; Jolly 1998; Weitz 2001). However, for the purposes of description here, I refer to accommodation and resistance in turn.

Accommodation relates to the passivity and docility referred to by Foucault thus preventing disturbance of power/knowledge relationships (Street 1992). However, Foucault does not relate this docility to subordination to a dominant ideology in the way that others do; for example Kirkham (1999). Kirkham describes the sense of 'helplessness', 'low expectations', 'acceptance of the status quo' and 'muteness' (737) experienced by midwives in relation to the dominant UK hospital-based maternity service culture. I adopt Kirkham's (1999) position, in that I believe that dominant ideologies do indeed provide a base for subordination of individuals.

Resistance contrasts with accommodation and takes two forms. First, passive resistance involves simply disregarding authoritative and public knowledges, or ignoring or modifying guidelines, policies or instructions (Street 1992; Hutchinson 1990). Active resistance, on the other hand, involves acting in a manner that is more liberating either for the individual or for others. This may involve challenging an ideology, public knowledge or authority and associated guidelines, policies and instructions (Street 1992; Weitz 2001). As stated, the most effective way in which to engage in active resistance is through collective action and challenge (Freire 1972; Burman 1992; Street 1992; Stanley and Wise 1993). This powerful form of resistance, that in turn yields transformation and emancipatory change, differs fundamentally from the Foucauldian concept of resistance located in the body, with the latter failing to deliver a political agenda (Freire 1972; Singer 1990; Burman 1992; Stanley and Wise 1993; Shildrik 1997; Standing 1998). As Burman (1992) states, from a feminist perspective, 'however much we deconstruct, comment on, take apart, we are still, *unlike* the deconstructionists, committed to putting something in its place' (50).

Clearly, while Foucault's theory provides important insights regarding power and its various manifestations, it also has limitations with regard to its relativity and lack of transformative potential. I return in the ensuing chapters to the issues raised here in relation to the data.

## Conducting the ethnographic study

I selected an ethnographic approach for the study to enable me to see and hear what was happening in order to provide a depth of understanding I did not feel I could achieve from simply conducting interviews with women. Ethnography originates from anthropology and is therefore informed and infused by the notion of culture. As Aamodt states:

> Ethnography is a way of collecting, describing and analysing the ways in which human beings categorise the meaning of their world [...]. It attempts to learn what knowledge people use to interpret experience and mould their behaviour within the context of their culturally constituted environment.
>
> (Aamodt 1991: 41)

Spradley (1980) refers to two levels of cultural knowledge: 'explicit' and 'tacit' (7). To recap, tacit knowledge refers to a knowledge that remains largely outside our immediate awareness, and explicit knowledge relates to a form of knowledge that people may communicate about with a relative ease. Spradley argues that what we see represents 'only the thin surface of a deep lake. Beneath the surface, hidden from view, lies a vast reservoir of *cultural knowledge*' (6). Ethnography aims to study both levels of knowledge. To study the latter the ethnographer must 'make inferences about what people know by listening carefully to what they say, by observing their behaviour, and by studying artefacts and their use' (Spradley 1980: 11). In this way, the ethnographer observes behaviour but moves beyond this to enquire about the meaning of the observed behaviour. To achieve this level of understanding of a given culture requires participating in people's lives over a considerable period of time, watching what happens, listening to what is said and asking questions (Hammersley and Atkinson 1995).

Hammersley and Atkinson (1995) chart ethnography's journey from a more descriptive and naturalistic discipline to embracing other theoretical perspectives ranging from interpretevism, critical inquiry, feminism and postmodernism. In its naturalistic form, ethnography rejected positivism which had previously dominated in the early twentieth century by emphasising that human behaviour was 'continually constructed and reconstructed' (8). However, the naturalistic approach to ethnography itself came under criticism in that it attempted to understand social phenomena as objects, existing independently of the researcher, that could be described and even explained in some literal fashion; this is akin to positivism.

I agree with this criticism in that, as Hammersley and Atkinson (1995) state, people construct their social world through their interpretations of it and their actions are then based on these interpretations. While these interpretations and actions reflect the underlying culture, they are not simply dictated by it. This view also requires an acknowledgement that the ethnographer's interpretations are influenced by her/his own culture (Spradley 1980). As Boyle (1994) asserts, ethnography is contextual and reflexive, emphasising the importance of context in understanding events and meanings, and taking into account the effects of the researcher and the research strategy on findings. It therefore combines the perspectives of both the participant and the researcher. It becomes clear that, as Hammersley and Atkinson (1995) assert, once the ethnographer him- or herself is seen in any way to be involved in constructing, there is incompatibility with the assumptions that underpin naturalistic ethnography. They argue that given the reflexivity required within social inquiry, it needs to be recognised that ethnographers indeed construct their descriptions of the social world rather than those accounts simply mirroring a reality.

Some ethnographers go further and embrace postmodernist or post-structuralist perspectives. Hastrup (1995) eloquently takes her readers on ethnography's journey through naturalism, interpretevism and finally postmodernism. She explodes the assumptions of early anthropologists by bringing the postmodern debate into the arena. She then arrives at a middle position in which she acknowledges that there is a place for ethnographic theories, arguing for a balance between relativity and realism. She presses for a firm move away from emphasis upon 'complete disengagement from the world' and its 'instrumental stance towards it' (173). On the other hand, she acknowledges that any interpretation cannot be entirely subjective because meaning must in some way be shared for it to contain meaning at all, thus reasserting that the explicit process of enculturation is still the cornerstone.

Clearly, the ethnographic approach may vary considerably according to the ethnographer's perspective and its resultant influence throughout the research process. Hammersley and Atkinson (1995) describe two key ways in which critical perspectives, to include feminism, have challenged traditional ethnography. There is critique first of the extent to which the political agenda influences the researcher and second of the extent to which ethnography is utilised to influence political and emancipatory change. Bibeau (1988), for example, stresses the 'powerful theoretical trend that stresses the importance of context, history and praxis in the interpretation of cultural codes'. This 'embraces the concepts of Foucault, Dumont, Gramsci, Bordieu and the neo-Marxists' (402). Thomas further elaborates, describing critical ethnography as a:

> type of reflection that examines culture, knowledge and action. It expands our horizons for choice and widens our experiential capacity to see, hear and feel. It deepens and sharpens ethical commitments by forcing us to develop and act upon value commitments in the context of political agendas. Critical ethnographers describe, analyze, and open to scrutiny otherwise hidden agendas, power centres, and assumptions that inhibit, repress, and constrain.
>
> (Thomas 1993: 3)

Thomas further argues that:

> The term *critical* describes both an activity and an ideology. As social activity, critical thinking implies a call to action that may range from modest rethinking of comfortable thoughts to more direct engagement that includes political activism. As ideology, critical thinking provides a shared body of principles about the relationship among knowledge, its consequences, and scholars' obligations to society.
>
> (Thomas 1993: 17)

These definitions point to the centrality of ideology, power and control in the research process, analysis and theoretical conceptualisations. However, I agree with Hammersley and Atkinson (1995) in their emphasis upon the need for balance between the impactless ethnography which allows the 'world to burn' and the ethnography which is underpinned by a clear political agenda (20). The latter may lead to a filtering out of information, thereby simply corroborating the political point-making, with resulting compromise of the data. To maintain this balance, I subjected the data presented in this book to several readings, endeavouring to represent the experiences and voices of the participants in combination with ideological critique.

I adopted an ethnographic approach, i.e. a topic-orientated ethnography that focused upon a specific aspect of activity within a given community (Spradley 1980), in this case women's experiences of breastfeeding on postnatal wards. The ethnographic study involved long periods of observation of activities on the postnatal wards, with particular reference to interactions between midwives and breastfeeding women. The observations were supplemented by interviews with both midwives and mothers. As Hammersley and Atkinson (1995) state, the two methods are mutually enhancing, in that what is seen informs what is asked about, and what is heard at interview informs what is looked for. Observation also enabled me to become aware of culturally learnt behaviour that may not be articulated at interview because much of the participants' cultural knowledge is tacit (Spradley 1980). This emphasis on describing what people do as well as believe is fundamental to ethnography (Brink and Edgecombe 2003).

## Settings and participants

The study was conducted between 2000 and 2004. I selected two maternity units, named hereafter as site one and two, in the north of England. The sites were different in some ways but the research was not set up as a comparative ethnographic study. Rather, two sites were selected to give depth to the study. Site one was a large consultant-led maternity unit in a city, with a high Caesarean-section rate reflecting its medicalised culture. The maternity unit was surrounded by a diverse range of areas in terms of the socio-economic status of the occupants. The unit served a predominantly white population but also served women of South Asian origin, most being second and third generation. The unit had two wards that provided for a mixture of ante and postnatal women. The two wards, named here as A and B, contained four-bedded rooms that opened into a central corridor, with a central 'station' running along the length of the corridor providing visibility to the open-plan rooms. This 'station' was rarely used by midwives as they tended to write their notes on women's bedside tables. There were also several side wards.

Site two was a smaller, less medicalised consultant-led maternity unit in a small town. The unit supported the local town and several large villages. There was one ward for ante and postnatal women and this was divided into four-bedded rooms and several side wards. Each room was separated from the corridor by a door that was usually closed. The community served was predominantly white. The populations served by both sites one and two were varied in terms of the socio-economic occupational status of service users, but both had high levels of unemployment, socio-economic deprivation and teenage pregnancy. On both sites hospital stay was normally twenty-four hours for multiparous women, three days for primiparous women and five days for women who had had a Caesarean section. Neither hospital was engaged with or working towards the Baby Friendly Hospital Initiative.

Sixty-one postnatal women participated in the study, having provided written consent, and seven women did not wish to participate. I included women who were admitted to the postnatal ward who had initiated breastfeeding and were able to communicate in written and verbal English. I excluded women whose babies were being cared for on the neonatal unit, women with serious obstetric, medical or emotional complications following childbirth, and women who did not wish to participate. Forty-eight of the participating women gave birth vaginally, eleven being instrumentally assisted. Thirteen women had a Caesarean section. Forty women were primiparous and twenty-one multiparous. Five women were Asian and fifty-six White, as defined by the UK Office of National Statistics classification (Hamlyn *et al.* 2002). The women represented a range from higher to lower socio-economic occupational groupings and ages seventeen to forty-two. These demographic profiles were broadly representative of the two local communities.

Thirty-nine midwives participated. None of the midwives refused to participate but they were often too busy to be interviewed. The midwives ranged from ages twenty-three to fifty-four and from newly qualified to over twenty-five years of experience. Thirty-eight of the midwives were female and one was male. One midwife was Asian and thirty-eight were white.

The study involved long periods of observation of activities in the postnatal wards, to include interactions between midwives and breastfeeding women. Participant observation was conducted for ninety-seven encounters between midwives and postnatal women during which breastfeeding was discussed. In addition, 106 focused interviews were carried out with postnatal women and thirty-seven with midwives. A tape recorder was utilised where appropriate and when permission from all parties was obtained.

## Observing

One of the decisions I had to make before entering the field was how to conduct the observations and to what extent I would be a participant or non-participant. Spradley (1980) describes all ethnographic observation as participant, in that the researcher is a part of the social situation. Hammersley and Atkinson (1995) likewise assert, 'there is a sense in which all social research takes the form of participant observation: it involves participating in the social world, in whatever role and reflecting on the products of that participation' (17).

Spradley (1980) refers to four levels of participation ranging from 'low' engagement to 'high' engagement (58). First, 'passive participation' involves the ethnographer being present at the scene but without interacting or participating with those s/he is observing; for example standing at a bus stop. 'Moderate participation' involves maintaining a balance between participation and observation. This may involve fluctuating between simply observing and participating in some ways. The third level that Spradley refers to is 'active participation'; this involves doing what the people in the study situation do to gain insight into the cultural codes and rules for behaviour. The final stage involves 'complete participation' when the researcher tends to already be a member of the group/situation to be studied.

On site one, I based myself at the 'station' enabling me to view the open-plan rooms. I was then able to 'move in' to observe a particular mother and midwife more closely when appropriate. On other occasions I based myself in a four-bedded room, when I wanted to focus upon one or two women in more depth, or when a mother declined to be observed in another room, making sitting at the 'station' unethical. On site two, I observed activities from within the rooms as they were self-contained. On a few occasions, I shadowed a midwife for the shift or session but this was more difficult due to the fragmented nature of their work. My level of participation was therefore 'moderate' (Spradley 1980: 58), but fluctuated between levels of activity, being more intensive when sitting in a room, and even more so when sitting behind curtains with a mother and midwife.

I sampled early, late and night periods of working, sometimes as single days and other times in blocks of two to five days. Periods of observation lasted approximately three to five hours during the day and eleven hours at night. My earlier observations were more general, with the 'station' being an ideal place to sit on site one. Spradley (1980) recommends a broad approach to the initial stages of ethnographic observations. This involved conducting 'descriptive observations'. These were more general observations guided by a nine-dimension framework for informing data collection:

1    Space: the physical place or places, i.e. ward layout, geography, nursery.
2    Actor: the people involved, i.e. the mothers and midwives.
3    Activity: a set of related acts people do; for example the postnatal examination or specific support with breastfeeding.

4   Object: the physical things that are present.
5   Act: single actions that people do.
6   Event: a set of related activities that people carry out.
7   Time: the sequencing that takes place over time.
8   Goal: the things people are trying to accomplish.
9   Feeling: the emotions felt and expressed.

(Spradley 1980: 78)

As the ethnographic research got underway I spent more time making 'focused observations' (Spradley 1980: 128). These involved focusing down to elicit more specific aspects of cultural meaning, such as the nature of the support offered to women when they requested assistance with, or information about, breastfeeding. Finally, I engaged in 'selective observations' involving a narrowing of the focus further to look for differences among specific cultural categories (Spradley 1980: 128). These required careful planning of very specific aspects to be observed. I conducted selective observations in response to the development of early theory and the need to test out my theorising and assumptions; for example I deliberately sought to observe the activities of a midwife whose approach was discrepant from that of previous midwives I had observed. This progressive focusing during data collection is also described by Hammersley and Atkinson (1995) as a gradual shift from describing social events and processes towards developing and testing theories. This included, as stated, searching for and focusing upon cases which would confirm or refute my early theorising.

I used a hand-held tape recorder to record interactions and interviews where possible, unless either mother or midwife refused permission. However, the spontaneous nature of some of the interactions did not lend themselves to me asking for permission, requiring note-taking instead. In all cases I took extensive notes as after the first few transcriptions I realised that some of the recordings were inaudible due to babies crying loudly, sudden lowering of voices or turning of heads away from the recorder. I noticed that when the midwife was actually assisting the mother to breastfeed, she would lean forwards and lower her voice to avoid disrupting the mother and baby's efforts. This meant that when I replayed the tape there would often be parts that were inaudible.

### Interviewing

Where possible I interviewed women folllowing an interaction but this was necessarily very flexible as women might then be involved in other activities. The interviews were flexibly guided by the specific context of each situation and the nature of preceding events and I therefore refer to them as 'focused'. They helped to clarify issues related to the interaction and included questions such as 'How has this discussion/encounter with the midwife influenced you with regard to breastfeeding?' Although I had an agenda I took care to remain open and flexible to issues raised spontaneously by women.

My initial intention was to focus upon interactions when carrying out subsequent interviews. However, when I approached women a second time, I found that they were more interested in talking about their experience since I last saw them, which in some cases was the day before. I also found that I was not always seeing regular interactions around breastfeeding and therefore I decided to follow some women through, where possible, for two to three days of their stay, in one case five days. In these situations I commonly asked, 'How do you feel about breastfeeding today?' and 'Tell me about your experiences of breastfeeding since I last saw you'. In most interviews the following issues were covered at some point: reason(s) for deciding to breastfeed; what type of support she had had with breastfeeding so far; intentions regarding breastfeeding after discharge from hospital; previous experience of breastfeeding (if multiparous).

Again, I progressively focused during data collection (Hammersley and Atkinson 1995) with individual women but also, as the study progressed, in order to test out my early theorising. I avoided imposing a priori categories during the early periods of data collection but as categories emerged they were incorporated into later interviews; for example it became evident that plans for the future influenced ways of negotiating the hospital breastfeeding experience. I therefore carefully sought out further data on this relationship. At all times, as recommended by May (1991), I endeavoured to flexibly achieve a balance between eliciting individual stories while ensuring enough consistency to allow for comparison between participants.

I asked women if they would like to talk to me in a private place with their baby with them, as there was usually an empty side room or day room. However, most preferred to talk by the bedside and due to the considerable volume of background noise these conversations were usually inaudible to others. In all cases I waited until the midwife had moved on to another room if I was asking women about a specific interaction. The discussions tended to be quite intermittent due to the baby waking or a midwife approaching. I taped interviews when permission was given but also took notes due to background noise and possible loss of data.

When it came to interviewing midwives, their extreme busyness meant that they were often unavailable to be interviewed in a quiet room for any length of time. Breaks were scarce and at the end of the 'shift' they wanted to get home, so opportunities were very limited. The most common ways in which midwives allowed me to elicit their views was by them initiating contact. This usually involved them coming up to me at the 'station' on site one or a quiet room on site two and talking to me, often rather vaguely, about an interaction but then moving swiftly on to provide me with contextual detail about the 'system'. This provided me with broader contextual detail about the ways that the culture within which they were working impinged upon them, influenced the women 'passing through' and impeded them in providing support for breastfeeding women. On these occasions I simply took notes, as to suggest tape-recording would, I felt, stifle the spontaneous nature of the discussions.

Although I had not anticipated the way in which midwives would direct the place, format and content of the conversations with me, the 'critical' nature of their comments assisted me in emphasising the influence of structure over agency for midwives, and the political over the personal, an essential facet of a critical study. This participant-led agenda shift was also described by Menzies (1970) in her classic organisational study of nursing. Despite her aim of developing new methods in nursing organisation, her focus was shifted by the nurses' repeated reference to their 'tension, distress and anxiety' (3).

### Ethical issues

I gained ethical approval for the study from the two relevant research ethics committees and the approved procedures were followed with regard to access, consent and participant autonomy. Access to the wards in which the study took place was granted by the head of midwifery on each site. I informed managers and staff about the study through the cascade management systems. I placed a notice about the study on view on each ward with contact details for any staff queries. I informed the midwife in charge of the ward prior to and on commencement of each observational period. Each time I commenced a period of observation I provided information sheets to all midwifery staff during the report time. I also informed midwives about the study, verbally indicating that they could choose not to participate or opt out at any stage during the observational period if they did not wish to be observed.

I approached the postnatal women who met the inclusion criteria at the commencement of each observational period or on their arrival to the ward. I informed them about the study and provided them with written information. After thirty minutes or longer I approached them again and invited them to participate. I asked if they had any further questions and then requested that they sign a consent form if willing to participate. I clarified that they could opt out at any stage or for any particular situation and that there would be no compromise to their care if they preferred not to participate. At all stages I protected participant autonomy and confidentiality. Pseudonyms are utilised next to the participant numbers (P for postnatal woman, MW for midwife).

### 'Stepping into role' – reflecting on my presence in the field

Hammersley and Atkinson (1995) refer to two perceived identities of the researcher, the expert and the critic, which make the gatekeeper(s) uneasy, i.e. 'the expectation of critical surveillance' (79). The midwives were clearly aware of my presence in the field, particularly when I was 'sitting in' with the midwife and mother. However, I made it clear that I was not there to provide any clinical care or to express any specific opinions. At first I felt that a few of the midwives were somewhat self-conscious and aimed to 'perform' well, making frequent eye contact with me to monitor my reaction. However, as time elapsed and it became clear to these midwives that I was not there to interact with them I found that they habituated to my presence and appeared not to be performing on my behalf. This stemmed partly from their obvious preoccupation with more pressing and concerning issues than someone observing them.

The 'Hawthorne effect' may have manifested. This relates to the effect of being studied upon those being studied, with knowledge of the study possibly influencing behaviour (Bowling 1997). In this study I have to acknowledge that support for breastfeeding women may have improved because of my presence. As the encounters and support (or lack of it) I observed still left considerable room for criticism I felt that any attempted improvements due to my presence did not fundamentally compromise the extent to which I was able to critique the situation. I also recognise my presence in the situation as an inevitable part of the construction of the social situation that should be exploited in a reflexive manner (Hammersley and Atkinson 1995).

I had to carefully reflect on the influence of my own history as both a midwife and a mother in order to avoid ignoring aspects of the environment that I had become familiar with in the past. As Hammersley and Atkinson (1995) warn, it is crucial to avoid the 'comfortable sense of being at home' with its associated risk of impeding one's ability to see and hear critically (115). They refer to the rhetoric around research legitimacy with some arguing that the 'insider' has exclusive rights, and others that the 'outsider' is better equipped. I felt that I was neither – rather, somewhere in the middle. I was maintaining a 'marginal position', i.e. a point between familiarity and strangeness (Hammersley and Atkinson 1995: 109–110). One example of something that I became acutely aware of, which I had habituated to when working in a maternity unit, was the intensity of the background noise. One of the profound ironies of being in the ethnographic role was that it enabled me to engage in a level of listening to women and understanding their situations that was often impossible for the midwives to achieve.

Freire (1972) states that 'reflection – true reflection – leads to action' (41). Reflexivity was crucial to this critical ethnographic study and involved a rejection of the bracketed ethnography and acknowledgement that I am inevitably influenced by my socio-cultural background and personal, political and intellectual values and beliefs (Stanley and Wise 1993; Hammersley and Atkinson 1995; Mauthner and Doucet 1998). As Mauthner and Doucet (1998) state, a 'profound level of self-awareness' is needed to 'capture the perspectives through which we view the world' and the 'filters through which we experience the world' (122). They recognise that being reflexive about data analysis involves locating oneself socially in relation to the researched, paying attention to one's emotional responses to the participants and examining how one makes theoretical interpretations (Mauthner and Doucet 1998).

Crucial to the critical ethnographic study was a constant reflection on power issues related to the actual research. Alldred (1998) cautions that power may operate through the language we use with its inevitable hegemonic cultural basis, through our position as a researcher, and our relationship with our participants. I needed to be constantly aware of the ways in which the researched might perceive me and how this would influence their responses to me. I have also reflected upon the power inherent in representing others. Standing (1998) argues that in representing others' perspectives, the relationship is inevitably one of unequal power because the researcher decides which parts of the data, interviews and women's words to present and which to omit and how to represent the findings. This challenged me throughout the entire process of the research.

I was ever conscious of the dilemmas in seeking to explore privately based knowledges and personal understandings and then reconstituting and presenting them in academic language in the public domain (Edwards and Ribbens 1998). In this way I felt that I was extending the dominance of publicly based knowledge and 'colluding in its intrusion into every nook and cranny of social life' (Edwards and Ribbens 1998: 13). However, without some form of collective representation these private knowledges would remain hidden, and the ways in which women may be struggling to carry out marginal, culturally ambiguous, embodied activities in a public domain would be largely invisible. Standing (1998) sums up the dilemma in representing women:

> One of our roles is to translate between the private world of women and the public world of academia, politics and policy. The dilemma remains of how we do this without reinforcing the stereotypes and cultural constructions we are challenging.
>
> (Standing 1998: 193)

### Analysis

Analysis of the data was cyclical, involving the discovery of new questions during the field work, which in turn guided my ongoing data collection through a process of iterative, concurrent data collection and analysis (Hammersley and Atkinson 1995). I transcribed the interview and observational data and I then developed basic, organising and global themes utilising thematic networks analysis (Attride-Stirling 2001). To support a critical analysis, I conducted further readings of the transcripts to identify issues related to ideology, power and control (Thomas 1993). Each global theme constituted a 'core, principle metaphor' that encapsulated the main point of the text (Attride-Stirling 2001: 393). I carried out a constant process of refinement and verification of the networks throughout the research process until no further basic themes emerged, there was no further movement of the themes, and the relationship between the themes was well established. Grounded theorists refer to this as 'theoretical saturation' (Strauss and Corbin 1990: 188).

My actions and interpretations throughout the research process were guided by the need to maximise the trustworthiness of the research. The process of concurrent data collection and analysis, with progressive focusing and seeking out discrepant cases, assisted me in gaining depth in the theoretical process (Spradley

1980; Hammersley and Atkinson 1995). Periods away from the field enabled me to engage in deep reflection upon the developing analytical themes. I obtained respondent validation (Appleton 1995) from the women who were interviewed on more than one occasion by presenting them verbally with key issues that they had highlighted the day before, during the interview, and asking whether or not they felt that these were for them the key issues. Throughout the research process I made my decision trail and thematic analysis transparent through peer review (Koch 1994).

## First impressions – the end of the medical production line

The hospital cultures were bureacratic with a production-line ethos, hierarchical structure and unpredictable, time-constrained working conditions for midwives and related staff. The experience for women was largely of a medical nature and encounters reflected the sub-culture from which they emanated. Both units were medicalised and becoming increasingly so with Caesarean-section rates rising year by year. As I observed the activities on the wards, I developed an overwhelming sense that I was at the end of a medical production line. The maternity hospital has been described as a 'conveyor belt' by Kirkham (1993: 6), but the sense of being at the final stage of that system was powerful as I situated myself within the postnatal ward culture. I wrote:

> My sense is one of being at the end of a fast medical conveyor belt. The women are often exhausted, stressed, and sedated. They are plunged into an unfamiliar setting, bombarded by a series of interactions with strangers and their spatial boundaries are constantly being invaded. Women who have had a Caesarean Section, even if under spinal anaesthetic but especially if under general anaesthetic, spend the first day unable to do much for themselves. They are immobilised and dependent on the midwives for 12–24 hours. There is an actual and symbolic relinquishing of autonomy for the final stop in the hospital.
>
> (Field notes)

The midwives always seemed to be very busy; this is now recognised as a frequent situation in the UK maternity services (Kirkham 1999; Kirkham and Stapleton 2001b). There appeared to be two major constraints upon midwives, first the powerful effects of linear time, as they were tied into a system in which their daily work centred upon urgency, meeting deadlines and literally racing against time. Midwives frequently commented upon the extreme busyness of the wards; for example:

> There isn't the time needed to help women, let alone give them appropriate breastfeeding support ... you can't do that when you're busy. You might have

several antenatals, an early labourer, post sections and we're even the over spill for gynae ... You just can't do it.

(Virginia, MW20)

Midwives' activities appeared to centre around saving time and using time efficiently, as also observed in related ethnographies (Street 1992; Kirkham and Stapleton 2001a; Stapleton *et al.* 2002b; Varcoe *et al.* 2003). However, their way of working was indeed far from efficient, based on the second major constraint, unpredictability. Unpredictability was created on both sites by the work patterns of midwives who could be called to delivery suite, theatre or antenatal clinic when needed, at a moment's notice. A midwife could come on to the ward and then go to clinic an hour and a half later for the reminder of the morning. This created anxiety and insecurity and led to a philosophy of needing to get the work done on the ward in case circumstances dramatically changed and the staff were suddenly depleted. Emergencies could arise at any time particularly with the antenatal women, creating more unpredictability. This situation contributed to a rushed, chaotic and fragmented approach to care as described by others (Ball 1994; Kirkham 1999; Kirkham and Stapleton 2000; Ball *et al.* 2002).

The midwives referred to the lack of control over working conditions, inability to get to know women, inflexibility and insecurity created by the organisational culture:

The main problem is never knowing when you might be moved ... can you really get to know anyone when you may be shifted off at a moment's notice. I mean some staff can be working on the ward, clinic, delivery and theatre all in one day. On top of that there aren't enough staff and therefore we can only try to give breastfeeding advice but often that's not enough.

(June, MW5)

Linda referred to the unpredictability of the working situation that reflected the super-valuation of the delivery suite:

The difficulty with this ward is that you can start off with only one room and an hour later you could have the whole ward. So you can't just take your time because you don't know when someone will be moved to delivery.

(MW32)

Women were inevitably influenced by the ways in which midwives were working, as illustrated by Helen:

They do seem to be so busy and understaffed. You have to catch people when you can, but it is not always the right timing, but when they have come they've been very helpful. I'd like to have someone checking to see that I'm doing all right ... The staff are rushing around. They are really helpful, but it can take a long time to get a little job done ... There's emergencies going on, and you don't feel that your request for help with something like breastfeeding is important enough to bother them with.

(Helen, P35 – on a very busy night)

Helen's comments resonate with those of others who describe postnatal care as the 'Cinderella' of the maternity service, reflecting its low position in the techno-medical hierarchy and its impoverished status in terms of resources and staffing (Ball 1994; Garcia *et al.* 1998; Anderson and Podkolinski 2000; McCourt and Percival 2000; Royal College of Midwives 2000a, 2000b; Singh and Newburn 2000). As Edwards (2000) states, 'the medical model, as a dominant ideology, has imposed its own structures and policies to manage birth and govern the distribution of resources in maternity services in ways that profoundly affect relationships between women and midwives' (61).

Not only were midwives under immense temporal pressures but they were also restricted spatially in many ways. It was often difficult for them to leave the ward due to lack of staff and the need to be around for emergencies. This restriction is an additional source of stress (Street 1992; Halford and Leonard 2003). Midwives powerfully illustrated their dissatisfaction with the 'system' by their actions and body language as they passed me. They often let out a loud 'sigh' and made comments indicating their relief at completing aspects of their work, surviving the shift and going off duty soon. The system, as I observed it, appeared to preclude any sense of meaningful relationships developing between midwives and women. Neither midwives nor mothers had any real influence regarding who they encountered in hospital. The ways in which midwives coped with 'caring' within this environment and the ways in which it impacted upon postnatal women are returned to, in depth, in Chapter 5. In the next chapter I turn to women's experiences of breastfeeding as labour.

# Chapter 4

# 'It's so demanding'

## Breastfeeding as labour

## Introduction

In this chapter I draw upon notions of labouring bodies to theorise women's perceptions of their role as breast-milk producers and deliverers and the demanding nature of this role. I utilise the industrial metaphor 'supplying' to illustrate the ways in which women conceptualised and negotiated this role with all of its inherent uncertainties. I then discuss the ways in which women experienced breastfeeding as physically and emotionally 'demanding' in terms of their temporal and bodily boundaries. I highlight the ways in which women, with their central preoccupation with supplying and demanding, sought ways in which to cope with and control the unpredictability of their bodily experiences of breastfeeding and the activities of their babies.

## Providing breast milk

### Doing what is right

Just as the language around labour is medical, in the sense that it emphasises measurable progress rather than the experiences of women (Downe and Dykes in press), so the language around breastfeeding currently centres upon its health benefits and its success in terms of delivery to the baby, duration and exclusivity. When I asked women about their reasons for deciding to breastfeed, few referred to breastfeeding as something to be experienced for mother and baby. There was a sense in which they might see a personal experience perspective as appearing to be self-indulgent, departing from the required selflessness of the ideal mother. The reasons women gave for breastfeeding were closely aligned with the strong current biomedical emphasis on the health benefits of breast milk. The women's reference to the health benefits was often made in a very automatic way, as if giving me the required answer. Women appeared to see breastfeeding as the 'correct' behaviour, a standardised ideal and as a one-way, non-reciprocal transmission of health to their baby, via the medium of breast milk. As Shaw (2003) states, 'as an expression of corporeal generosity between mother and child, the transferring of nourishment from mother to infant is conventionally identified as a natural, non-contractual, bio-physiological act' (68).

What alarmed me was the dispassionate manner in which the decision to breastfeed was expressed. Women appeared to have internalised the public discourse that 'breast is best', to such an extent that they were no longer expressing their 'feeling voices' (Ribbens 1998: 35). Ribbens refers to the replacement of 'feeling voices' by 'moral voices', be they 'pragmatic', 'puritanical', 'idealistic' or 'watch for the future' (35). Sophie, when asked why she decided to breastfeed, illustrated this in her impersonal use of institutional language:

> Um ... just because of everything you read is breast is best ... you know ... helps you ... helps your baby. It does help you lose your weight but it's best for babies... more settled babies ... and obviously everything's in breast milk but er ... it's good for them ... so breast is best.
>
> (P61)

By far the main reason given for breastfeeding by women, as reported by others (Schmied 1998; Murphy 1999, 2000; Schmied *et al.* 2001), was that breast milk conferred health benefits on the baby due to its superior nature deriving from its immunological and nutritional factors; for example, 'it's better for the baby, more nutrients and it's balanced and there's everything there that they need'(Jackie, P33); 'for her sake really as much as anything, for giving antibodies and things, especially in the first few weeks' (Andrea, P54). The 'breast milk is natural' discourse was very strong; for example:

> I mean I think it's obviously natural with immunity things and everything else, and um, I just think if it wasn't produced (*laughs*), there's a reason for everything isn't there, so um, that's the way nature intended, so stick with it.
>
> (Barbara, P37)

A few women referred to bonding, usually in a rather matter-of-fact way, with little reference to intimacy: 'bonding; I'm doing it for bonding' (Bev, P2).

It is beyond the scope of this research to draw conclusions related to differences between Asian and white women, particularly as the South Asian women may have lived in the UK for most or all of their lives. However, it was striking that only one woman, from Gujarat, referred to intimacy, closeness and nurture, 'intimacy really is the main reason. I'm from India, from Gujarat ... People there breastfeed for about two years' (Usha, P36). This relational orientation represents a clear difference from the western biomedical conceptualisation of breast milk as a product important for its nutritional components (Van Esterik 1988). The absence of dichotomy between the baby's nutritional and emotional needs within some traditional communities is highlighted in anthropological studies; for example in Mali (Dettwyler 1987), Papua New Guinea (Jenkins *et al.* 1984) and rural parts of the Indian sub-continent (Vincent 1999; Spiro 2006).

Women tended to see breastfeeding as being a part of the performance or project of good motherhood as referred to by others (Maclean 1989; Bottorff 1990; Blum 1993, 1999; Carter 1995; Schmied 1998; Murphy 1999; Schmied and Barclay 1999; Stearns 1999; Bartlett 2000; Pain et al. 2001; Wall 2001; Meyer and de Oliveira 2003; Shaw 2003). Indeed, they expressed the power and pressure of the 'breast is best' ideology upon their experience of new motherhood. Andrea talked about her previous experience as being one of pressure, guilt and failure to achieve her idealised notions of motherhood:

> I breast fed my little boy but not for very long ... I had very sore nipples and then I got mastitis, so I expressed for a while instead and then I finished breastfeeding when he was six or seven weeks. This time though coming into it I was thinking if it didn't work it didn't matter. Whereas when I had Tom I was so guilt ridden that I couldn't do it. It had been my fault and all that sort of business, so I've come into it a lot more relaxed this time ... There's a lot of pressure, there's a lot of expectations that you will breastfeed without problems, so when I had problems, I felt guilty as if it was my fault. I felt that there shouldn't be problems. You have this vision of perfection and the pressure builds up to do everything how it should be done.
>
> (P54)

Despite women's reiteration of the notion that breastfeeding was the 'natural ideal', women who were breastfeeding for the first time and some for a subsequent time tended to describe their early experiences as far from 'natural' or 'ideal'. There was a strong sense of dissonance between expectation and reality as described by others (Bowes and Domokos 1998; Schmied 1998; Dykes and Williams 1999; Hoddinott and Pill 2000; Mozingo et al. 2000; Pain et al. 2001; Hauck and Irurita 2003). The dissonance in this study between the expectation of a 'natural experience' and the reality left women with a sense of detachment from breastfeeding that they had difficulty expressing verbally. As Miller (1998) asserts in relation to mothering, 'it is not easy to give an account of experiencing something which does not resonate with the public story of becoming a mother, especially when the public assumption exists that all women naturally know how to mother' (61).

Shaw (2003) challenges the tendency to naturalise what may be perceived as bodily exchanges between social subjects who are engaged in a gift relationship; a notion which for some women brings with it feelings of risk and uncertainty. The discursive connection between 'good' mothering and naturalness is particularly strong, with breastfeeding being portrayed as a significant activity within the natural realm of women (Apple 1987; Schmied 1998; Leff et al. 1994; Carter 1995; Shaw 2003). It is then assumed that if breastfeeding is natural, it should be straightforward and simple. However, as Shaw (2003) again argues:

> The relation between maternal desires, one's identification as a 'good mother' and actual experiences of breastfeeding are not so straightforward. Bad experiences of breastfeeding – for whatever reason – may in fact induce or motivate women to distance themselves from disciplinary technologies and social norms and expectations they regard at odds with their own sensory understandings and dispositions.
>
> (Shaw 2003: 64)

The embedding of breastfeeding into notions of what women are and should become caused particular dissonance for women if breastfeeding became difficult. Kate expressed surprise at the challenge breastfeeding created: 'it looked quite um ... simple (*laughs*) um ... until you come to do it. Like I'm impatient, I thought she'd just take to it, because um ... it's natural and that' (P39). During an interview three days after her baby's birth, Chloe exemplified the feelings of dissonance between her notion of breastfeeding as natural and therefore simple and the reality of her actual experience:

> I think there's no such thing as getting it absolutely right from the first moment, because I think you have fairly high expectations of yourself ... You know, it's a new process and you can't expect it to be wonderful straight away and you know, not every baby's the same ... You know, things that I hadn't really thought of before ... it [the birth] all happened more quickly than I expected; I was at sea with everything. I think there's an expectation that you'll be able to do it and there's been a lot of medical attention, media attention and so on about breastfeeding being the best thing for your baby, and, you've got lots of sort of media posters downstairs on breastfeeding and that's the whole image that's conveyed, that this is something that you should be doing ... And I think if you had difficulty doing it then you'd probably feel as I felt yesterday – I'm not really adequate, you know ... I'm not doing this properly; I've failed somehow. I felt that about my labour as well, because I knew I wasn't pushing the way they wanted me to push, I didn't understand how to do it differently ... And it's that, I think, because there's such sort of emphasis on it, as being a process that is natural and instinctive, you think, yes it must be because people have been giving birth behind bushes for centuries and all sorts of things – it must be a natural thing to do. But if it doesn't come naturally to you then you feel like you've failed. I think it's that ... I mean I've never really entertained the possibility of it just not happening ... I think it's um, just you know ... obviously you have time to reflect on things when you're in hospital, you just think your life is sophisticated and so much influenced by technology, and then you're in a situation where you're expected to do something which, as I say, is sort of instinctive and back to your roots again, and you haven't been there for so long. You haven't done anything instinctive because you know you're part of this digital world and everything. It's really quite strange ... It reminds me of the Nigella Lawson

book, *How to be a Domestic Goddess?* It's a cookery book, but it's really ... I've only used one or two recipes out of it, but at the beginning of it she's sort of self-parodying really in terms of why she's chosen that title, you know sort of cooking a nice cake or something that's home made doesn't make you into a domestic goddess, but it makes you feel as though you're somebody who is actually providing in a different way than if you go out and do your pot noodle or whatever, and that's the sort of essence of it and um, that was what I was doing on Monday (*laughs*) when my waters broke ... But yes, I got some cakes at the end of it, but it's just a sort of bizarre feeling, that somebody's saying, you know have the freedom to do this rather than all the nouvelle cuisine sort of thing ...

(P50)

Chloe's reflections illustrate some of the confusing dilemmas for women between notions of naturalness and life in the 'digital age'. She felt strangely disconnected from her busy technologically dependent life as a teacher:

I mean our school is being inspected in February so the last few weeks have been about action planning and statistics and that sort of thing and you know I haven't got a clue now and to be honest I couldn't care less ... Oh well if we've not got that many fours at key stage two, who cares! It's strange ... your whole mentality just switches over, so it's quite nice to have left all that lap top business behind and just think, oh I can actually have a bit of time where I'm in touch with what, you know, life was like in a different age. I feel like going out and reading lots of Thomas Hardy novels. It's that feeling that perhaps none of all that really matters, you know, this is a new life and in the end she's going to hopefully survive all those government agendas and things and it's what goes on between you and the baby that's important.

Here Chloe illustrated the way in which her temporality altered from a pressured linear perspective to a more cyclical experience (Kahn 1989), an issue I return to later. Chloe's narrative powerfully illustrates the transformative experiences of pregnancy, birth, motherhood and breastfeeding and the potential for these processes to be disrupted by unrealistic expectations about what women 'should naturally achieve'. Women did not seem to be prepared for the uncertainty of early breastfeeding and indeed new motherhood – an issue I return to later with regard to women's experiences of demand feeding.

### Resisting the 'gaze'

Women's dissonance with regard to providing breast milk was potentiated by feelings of being under surveillance in hospital. In Chapter 1 I referred to Foucault's concept of surveillance that operates at various levels. First, he refers to 'hierarchical surveillance', i.e. by the disciplinary institution with the building being designed to accommodate a high level of scrutiny. Second, he refers to the 'normalising gaze' upon the body by medical personnel (1977: 170). He links the disciplinary regimes with the body and emphasises the power of medicine through its techniques of questioning, monitoring, watching, spying, searching out, palpating and bringing into the light to label what is normal and what is deviant (Foucault 1981). Rituals and techniques establish a power of normalisation over individuals (Foucault 1976, 1977, 1980, 1981). For Foucault (1977) normalisation is seen in 'the case' and the way in which it is 'described, judged, measured, compared with others' (191). In this way the medical gaze during the clinical encounter inscribes the body until eventually the individual will start to police, self-monitor and discipline her/his own body.

The forms of surveillance I observed provided a striking representation and indeed magnification of the ambiguous positions women are faced with when breastfeeding in western communities. Foucault's (1977) reference to the 'productive' yet 'subjected' body seems to be very appropriate to breastfeeding mothers who are expected to be productive – producing breast milk, but their bodies are also subjected to surveillance of their performance and to dominant and authoritative forms of knowledge (26). Indeed Foucault (1981) refers to breastfeeding as a 'dangerous period [...] saturated with prescriptions' (37). The concept of the gaze upon individual bodies and its self-regulating potential is highly relevant to the female body. As Shildrick (1997) argues:

> The gaze now cast over the subject body is that of the subject herself. What is demanded of her is that she should police her own body, and report in intricate detail its failure to meet standards of normalcy; that she should render herself, in effect transparent. At the same time the capillary processes of power reach even deeper into the body, multiplying here not desire but the norms of function/dysfunction. As with confession, everything must be told, not by coercive extraction, but 'freely' offered up to scrutiny.
>
> (49)

This is particularly relevant for women as they embark on breastfeeding. Breastfeeding on a postnatal ward presented, and indeed magnified, dilemmas for women at the very heart of dualistic discourses around culture and nature, public and private, maternal and sexual. The notion of 'natural', as Blum (1999) asserts, usually signals what is 'good, authentic, and untainted by social or human manipulation, and thus "natural" motherhood seems to belong outside the public realm' (13). However, as Martin (1987) states, 'women's bodily processes go with them everywhere, forcing them to juxtapose biology and culture' (200).

The 'mother as nurturing' versus 'woman as sexual' dualism was magnified for women in hospital. As stated, breastfeeding currently symbolises good mothering and, as Stearns (1999) argues, 'it is a visual performance of mothering with the maternal body at centre stage' (308). She refers to breastfeeding in public as 'transgressing the boundaries of both the good maternal body and woman-as-

(hetero)sexual object' with the sexual breast and maternal breast being required to be independent of each other as the 'meaning and place of women's breasts is contested' in western culture (310). The dissonance created for women by the blurring of boundaries between breastfeeding as a maternal activity and display of sexual breasts is highlighted in the literature (Van Esterik 1994; Carter 1995; Rodriguez-Frazier and Frazier 1995; Blum 1999; Stearns 1999; Hawkins and Heard 2001; Mahon-Daly and Andrews 2002). This dissonance may be increased by the embodied experience of breastfeeding as intimate, sensuous and erotic (Odent 1992; Rodriguez-Frazier and Frazier 1995; Shaw 2003). The leakiness of the body may potentiate dissonance as women contend with the additional dualism between breast milk as pure and life-giving and their secretions as a subversive corporeal manifestation of unboundedness (Spiro 1994, 2006; Britton 1997; Shildrick 1997; Bramwell 2001, Bartlett 2002).

Women tended to monitor and resist the male gaze by closing their curtains around themselves, 'I like the privacy while I'm feeding, ... you don't want an audience do you (*laughs*) and there are husbands and that' (*laughs*) (Corinne, P41). Corinne was also concerned about how the visitors would feel, 'I mean I don't want to feed in front of visitors, like I'm not bothered, but er, it puts them in an awkward position, like'. Stella referred to a similar concern about others viewing her body:

> Well, I just leave them (curtains) round cos I'm feeding all day. Like if any of my own relatives come and that like ... that doesn't bother me but um ... and like trying to get out of bed, it's not very lady-like really.
>
> (Stella, P46)

The careful negotiation of space and place in relation to breastfeeding that I observed has become a feature of women's breastfeeding experiences (Pain *et al.* 2001; Mahon-Daly and Andrews 2002). As Stearns states, 'women accomplish the breastfeeding of their children with constant vigilance to location, situation, and observer' (322). This negotiation does not simply occur in public places such as shopping areas, but may occur at home when visitors arrive.

High levels of visibility created problems for women when they were experiencing difficulties with breastfeeding. As stated, authoritative health knowledges, although unstable and shifting, exert a coercive power over women in that they bring with them an apparatus of institutional regulation and surveillance. The ways in which women accommodate, resist or disregard these knowledges and the related surveillance varies depending upon the context. I now provide one example of an authoritative knowledge, 'exclusive breastfeeding is best', to illustrate the connections between knowledge, power and surveillance and their influence upon women's experiences.

Few would argue with the value of exclusive breastfeeding for infant health on physiological and immunological grounds (WHO 2001, 2003; Kramer and Kakuma 2003). However, anthropological and historical literature sources illustrate the numerous ways in which women have combined breastfeeding with other forms of food and drink throughout recorded history and across the globe (Fildes 1986; Maher 1992a). This pattern continues in many western industrialised countries; for example in the UK the per centage of breastfeeding women using formula milk for their four-to-ten-week-old babies was 41 per cent in 2000. Only 25 per cent of mothers were exclusively breastfeeding at this stage in the survey (Hamlyn *et al.* 2002: 48). Despite this knowledge that many women breast and formula feed simultaneously, as Blum (1999) asserts (with regard to the US), there is now a public health discourse that presents the bottle-versus-breast decision as either-or absolutes. However, in many communities in the UK the breast or bottle option stands in contradiction to a cultural norm.

The issue of exclusive breastfeeding is very challenging. There is a clear need to reverse the earlier practice of giving almost all babies supplements, with or without parental consent, recognising that giving formula milk to breastfed babies is closely connected with early cessation of breastfeeding. There is also an imperative to counteract the exploitative role formula companies have played in demoting the practice of exclusive breastfeeding. However, women's accounts in this study illuminate some of the dilemmas created for women by their dissonance regarding authoritative knowledge about exclusive breastfeeding within a culture where this practice is far from the current norm. Anna illustrated her feelings of deviance, the ways in which she felt under surveillance and how she endeavoured to resist the 'gaze' when faced with breastfeeding difficulties and her desire to mix breast and bottlefeeding:

> It's drummed in at parent-craft, there are posters everywhere and books; breastfeeding is all rosy ... I mean you get pregnant and read all the magazines and books, like *Mother and Baby* and Miriam Stoppard. It is all a happy picture of breastfeeding, but when it comes down to it you've had pethidine, you're drowsy ... I feel a failure ... um ... The advice you get is like all or nothing ... There's nothing about bottle feeding, except ... 'how bad'. I want the best but bottle feeding can't be all that bad ... It becomes a really big thing like you've got to breastfeed. I've got my options open, but there's too much pressure to do one or the other. When I was shaking a bottle up this morning and the midwife went past I tried to hide it, because I felt naughty.
>
> (P1)

The staff appeared to give little explanation as to why exclusive breastfeeding was the optimum way of feeding, tending simply to restate that it was better for the baby. Any form of discussion about ways in which Anna might combine breastfeeding with bottle feeding, even in the short-term, was also strikingly absent even though this was clearly Anna's preference. Anna then decided before going home that she would exclusively bottle feed with infant formula. Indeed she discharged herself home and thus resisted what she saw as an authoritative 'gaze'. This resistance illustrates, as Ribbens (1998) comments, that women do exercise agency in their lives and do not simply accept some ideology per se. Nevertheless, little is known about the extent to which the idealised way of breastfeeding and the surveillance in place to monitor it may be internalised negatively by women who feel they cannot or do not want to meet the recommended standard.

## Supplying

While rigid practices of separating mothers from babies have been largely reversed, separation was ever present in this study in the way many of the women understood and experienced breastfeeding. Women commonly conceptually separated the act of nutrition from notions of nurture and relationality. They saw their breasts as functioning to make milk that they were required to deliver or transfer to the baby. However, they were deeply mistrusting of their body's ability to produce the 'correct' amount and the right quality of the product, breast milk, and they doubted their ability to deliver this to the baby. I use the words 'produce', and 'deliver', being fully aware of their metaphorical alignment with industry and the production line. As I discussed in Chapter 2, this language was, and indeed still is, highly evident in biomedical texts on breastfeeding. It also reflects the ways in which women appeared to understand and experience breastfeeding whilst still in hospital.

There has been considerable reference in the literature related to perceived 'insufficient milk' – a phenomenon that is reported in industrialised countries around the world (Hillervik-Lindquist 1991, 1992; Segura-Millan *et al.* 1994; Dykes and Williams 1999; Blyth *et al.* 2002; Dykes 2002, 2005a; Hamlyn *et al.* 2002; Cooke *et al.* 2003). It remains the most common reason why women in the UK discontinue breastfeeding and is a consistent feature of six quinquennial infant feeding reports (Martin 1978; Martin and Monk 1982; Martin and White 1988; White *et al.* 1992; Foster *et al.* 1997; Hamlyn *et al.* 2002). Cross-cultural anthropological studies illustrate that 'insufficient milk syndrome' is a phenomenon which predominates in cultures infiltrated by the western biomedical view that breast milk is primarily a product (Van Esterik 1988).

For women to express mistrust in their capabilities at such an early stage suggests that they have come to the experience of breastfeeding with many doubts. This relates, at least partially, to the dualistic and mechanistic representations of the body (Beekman 1977; Illich 1995; Hastrup 1995; Davis-Floyd and Dumit 1998) and in particular the defining discourses of femininity over the past two centuries in the west, which have assisted in constructing the female body as weak, defective and deeply untrustworthy (Oakley 1986; Martin 1987; Schwarz 1990; Kohler Reissman 1992; Davis-Floyd 1992, 1994; Duden 1993; Carter 1995; Shildrick 1997; Blum 1999). Superimposed upon this mistrust is the reinforcement of the tenets of the techno-medical paradigm during pregnancy, labour and birth. As Millard states in relation to women's births:

Women thus are made to conform to schedules, and the signals they receive from their own bodies are interpreted as irrelevant or misleading in contrast

> to measurements taken by machines and nurses. Women come to breastfeeding with a recent intense experience in ignoring their own bodily signals, which have been redefined as problems instead of guides to action.
>
> (Millard 1990: 212)

As I discussed in Chapter 1, the current 'seeing is believing' culture in the UK is exemplified during pregnancy, labour and birth, during which women become increasingly exposed to the notion of dependency upon visual verification and validation of embodied experiences (Duden 1993). Ironically, as the quest for visualisation has increased exponentially, the mother appears to have become increasingly invisible (Oakley 1986; Martin 1987; Duden 1993).

In relation to breastfeeding, in the west the focus is very much upon breastfeeding as a physical activity whose function is to provide nutrition for the baby. In essence, it is about breast milk feeding the physical body (Vincent 1999). Growth can be seen and measured as verification of the effectiveness of this process, with the mother being placed centre stage for any blame related to her baby failing to grow at the prescribed rate. Therefore, women are faced with a combination of feeling accountable for producing breast milk and performing appropriately to ensure effective delivery to the baby. At the same time their bodies are the subject of mistrust and are seen as in need of surveillance and management.

Oakley (1986) refers to an 'uneasy balance between a dependence on medical authority and the need to trust one's own knowledge of one's body' (238). The preoccupation with measurement of breast milk that developed with the general medicalisation of infant feeding at the turn of the twentieth century is still highly evident in today's biomedical literature. While the methods have become more sophisticated, the principles are the same. An example of the perpetuation of these principles may be seen in a description of the 'pros' and 'cons' of measurements, to include test weighing, isotope measurement, breast expression and the recent technique of computerised breast measurement (Cregan and Hartmann 1999). Here the authors discuss the measurement of rate of milk synthesis, breast storage capacity, degree of breast fullness and volume of milk removed.

As I discussed in Chapter 2, the aggressive global marketing of infant formula by powerful multinational corporations, and display of breast-milk substitute slogans in healthcare clinics, are also argued to have played a major role in the lack of cultural belief in the efficacy of breastfeeding (Palmer 1993; Sokol 1997; Dykes 2002). This was greatly assisted by the super-valuation of science and its associated developments to assist with modern ways of living. The bottle therefore represented liberation and formula milk represented the superiority of science (Apple 1987; Palmer 1993; Quandt 1995).

Breastfeeding in the UK is now seen very much as a learned skill. This relates to women entering their transition to motherhood, from an essentially bottle feeding culture, often having had little or no previous personal experience of breastfeeding and having little opportunity for vicarious experience, i.e. watching others (Hoddinott 1998; Hoddinott and Pill 1999a, 1999b; Dykes 2003). The lack of culturally acquired knowledge creates an opening for authoritative biomedical knowledge related to breastfeeding to predominate and a concomitant lack of confidence in breastfeeding. Women then become dependent upon health workers to provide them with support in the form of practical assistance, information and encouragement.

The global theme of 'supplying' encompasses two organising themes: 'production' of breast milk and 'delivery' to the baby, which I consider in turn.

### Production

Women appeared to conceptualise their breasts as potentially faulty machines; they used language such as, 'it's not working ... I'm not very confident because it's not working' (Annette, P58). The language Annette and other women used in relation to their concerns tended to objectify their breasts, illustrated by a striking lack of use of personal pronouns. Mahon-Daly and Andrews (2002) refer to this distancing from one's body and conceptual disconnection from one's breasts, particularly when the body does not appear to be functioning. Balsamo *et al.* (1992) likewise refer to the alienation of the self, the body and its products, which are experienced as outside the self when breastfeeding is problematic. One of the midwives, Virginia, illustrated women's lack of body confidence, making clear connections between birth and breastfeeding:

> The trouble is that women don't believe in themselves, in relation to their birth or breastfeeding. They don't think they can do it. Look at the section rates. They're nearly 25 per cent and they're increasing all the time. In my opinion there are too many inductions, then you get failure to progress, and then a section. Then if you've had a previous emergency section, you end up choosing an elective section next time so it's bound to go up and up. Women don't believe they can manage in labour and they don't believe they can breastfeed. Some of them – they just sit there (*Gestures arms out, chest out*), they don't have a clue; they're all tense, they've read all the books and they make it so complicated.
>
> (Virginia, MW20)

Women tended to discuss breastfeeding in relation to the contrasting certainty inherent in bottle feeding and being able to measure how much the baby was getting. Nadine felt that she could not measure intake because she was unable to visualise the quantity of breast milk being provided:

> It still worries me that I don't know how much she's taking ... (*laughs*) ... but they've told me not to worry about that so ... but I think it's purely because if you're giving a bottle you know ... you can actually physically see how much she's taken, whereas I know like it's demand feeding and they're only taking

what they want and what they need ... apparently ... but it's still ... you can't physically see it ... you can't see it and that's the worry.

(Nadine, P60)

Some women endeavoured to monitor their milk through visualisation by, for example, squeezing milk out:

I did get a bit worried though and I asked the midwife to come because when I squeezed to get a bit of milk, before I fed her, there was nothing there, and then she sucked for half an hour and when she came off she was crying.

(Sally, P40)

Jo saw linear time as a crude way of assessing the volume of breast milk taken by her baby. This was seen as inferior to the accuracy possible when measuring formula milk:

I'm worried if she's getting enough. You know with formula you can measure. With breast milk it's difficult to get an accurate amount, you can only go on time, but ... I suppose though, if she wanted more she would keep going?

(Jo, P45)

The above quotes reflect women's clear desire to measure breast milk in order to provide reassurance and validation that they had enough, as reported in other contexts (Leff *et al.* 1994; Kavanagh *et al.* 1995; Dykes and Williams 1999; Dykes 2002). This relates to a desire for predictability through quantification and the general feeling that to see is to know (Duden 1993). While in the field I inevitably heard midwives talking to women who were bottle feeding with infant formula. I am unable to report on this as data as neither the mothers nor midwives had consented to me using these encounters as data. However, as a general statement, I was particularly struck by the emphasis upon accurate measurement at every stage of the process, with too much or too little powder being portrayed as problematic and even dangerous, which indeed it can be when formula feeding. This stark contrast between the way in which women are expected to trust the process of breastfeeding for meeting their baby's entire nutritional needs and the scientific precision related to formula feeding illuminates one of the sources of dissonance for women. Demand feeding, with all its inherent irregularity and unpredictability, appeared to increase women's anxieties related to the adequacy of their milk; this is an issue I turn to later in this chapter.

The colostrum (early milk) phase appeared to be experienced as particularly uncertain for most women, who felt anxious that colostrum was insufficient for their baby, for example:

He's not getting much milk – only colostrum ... I mean ... you know ... he's feeding but you don't know how much they're getting because you can't see it coming, you know, because it's still only the colostrum.

(Corinne, P41)

Women anxiously awaited the arrival of the 'proper milk', as illustrated by Sandra (P34) who had breastfed for a few weeks with her first baby. She thought that feeling heavy breasts would reassure her that she had milk, in contrast to the lack of any tangible sign in relation to colostrum:

When he's not fed really like you just think, if you see other babies feeding you just worry that they're not getting enough food really, um ... but then everyone says he's all right and I mean he's not screaming or anything ... You can't see how much they are getting it's very strange because I know there's like colostrum; I know that's in there but you can't see it and sometimes you think; 'is there anything actually coming out?' (laughs). It's illogical really isn't it (laughs) ... it's that you can't see it. I mean I know once your milk comes in it's different again, cos you can feel your breast becoming heavy and solid and you can see it coming out, but right at the very very beginning ... I mean it's tangible then isn't it, whereas with colostrum you can only squeeze a tiny bit out.

(Sandra, P34)

Sandra's reference to food again illustrates the way in which women conceptualised breastfeeding primarily as a source of nutrition with little apparent emphasis upon relationship. Her sense of waiting for the next stage, for the milk to come in, reflects the general desire for linear progress to take place. Simonds (2002) refers to this conceptualising of reproductive experiences into reified time slices whose progression to the next stage is a mark of progress. This fracturing of procreative events, she argues, reflects the masculinist ideologies which permeate obstetric care.

A sense of progress was experienced when the milk came in:

They're [breasts] a lot harder now and there's definitely more come through because I can tell by the way he's sort of gulping more rather than just; it's the noise he makes I can tell he's taking more.

(Corinne, P41)

In spite of the waiting for the milk to come in, some women still tended to feel anxious thereafter:

His feeding has changed since my milk's come in – before he was feeding quite frequently, but now it's less often and not for so long ... I haven't got much confidence because I don't know whether he's getting enough or I don't like the fact that he's not feeding so regularly now. I think it's about your expectations isn't it, because when they're on the bottle you can see exactly how much they're getting ... I didn't really know what to expect.

(Harriet, P52)

### Delivery

Women were not only concerned about production but also delivery of the produced milk to the baby. Women sometimes expressed concerns related to the actual flow of breast milk from their bodies:

I don't feel ... you know ... that there was enough leaving my body, it's a weird sort of feeling, you want to give the baby the best start in life, but you're not sure.

(Chloe, P50)

This relates to the western expectation that milk will flow according to linear time constraints, as illustrated by Spiro's (1994, 2006) research with women who had moved to the UK from rural Gujarat who had not encountered this anxiety about milk flow in India. She argues that it relates to a loss of closeness to body rhythms in western societies and a loss of closeness between two bodies: that of the mother and that of the baby. Women also tended to be concerned that their milk might not actually be reaching their baby:

It's just knowing what's happening. You know she just gorges herself and then it's like coming out of her nose and everywhere, so you don't know if they're getting enough, like if it's coming out of there how do you know she's getting enough ... and the other thing, like yesterday, she fed at half past seven in the morning, but she'd been in that incubator so she was tired and cosy, and I had to wake her at ten to two and I was quite worried because I thought well ... she was feeding for up to an hour before that so there was like this big change in time and I just thought well ... is she not well? ... because obviously I had to wake her in the first place and secondly is that ten minutes enough for her when it's so rich?

(Jane, P12)

Jane appears to have conceptualised the changes in 'time' between feeds as indicative that all might not be well in terms of delivery to the baby. Women saw gaining confidence in the skill of breastfeeding as a primary goal in ensuring effective 'delivery' to the baby, 'I mean mainly at the moment, I want to be confident that I can do it' (Selina, P48). Women tended to state that they knew that breast milk was best but then felt that they needed to know what to do:

I'm confident knowing that it's the best for her, that's why I decided when I was pregnant to breastfeed her, but I want to feel confident with what I'm doing, you know, with what to do.

(Kate, P39)

Women tended to become anxious when the baby became discontented and unhappy, and this made them doubt their ability to deliver the 'product' effectively:

I was a bit stressed in the night – cos he was crying – you don't know what's wrong with them – you don't know if it's something that you've done, like you've not fed them enough or you're not doing it properly.

(Glynnis, P59)

Sam (P19) said, 'I'm not convinced I'm doing it right myself. The milk hasn't come through yet. It's still colostrum ... she just doesn't seem happy.' Her baby did not appear to be very effectively attached to her breast and she had very sore nipples, which probably contributed to the baby being unsettled. The associations between what women see as unsettled behaviours and their perceptions of insufficient milk are well established (Hill and Aldag 1991; Perez-Escamilla *et al.* 1994; Segura-Millan *et al.* 1994; Foster *et al.* 1997; Hamlyn *et al.* 2002) and, when related to ineffective patterns of breastfeeding, are likely to have a physiological basis (Woolridge 1995).

In contrast, women felt confident when their baby was settling between feeds. This enhanced their feeling that they were producing and delivering enough milk:

Up till now, I feel confident, just because she seems content on it and like as soon as she's had enough she just goes straight to sleep, um ... I mean it's early days so I don't know if it's going to stay like this or whether she's just behaving herself for now. But it gives me confidence to know that she's feeding and then she seems quite content after it.

(Millie, P43)

Women endeavoured to assess their milk transfer to the baby through various means, for example watching what comes out:

My only worry at the moment is that he passed a stool yesterday, he did his meconium and then he passed a normal stool but he hasn't since, so my worry is that, I mean, I hope he is getting what he needs because he seems to be sleeping afterwards, and he's content, but because nothing is coming out my fear is that he is just kind of suckling rather than well, you know, he's doing it for comfort rather than ... but I think he'd probably be crying and upset if he wasn't getting enough ... um ... I just assumed that with them having such little stomachs that it would just come straight through them.

(Alison, P38)

Women focused on using the 'correct' technique to deliver the milk and this led to preoccupation with, for example, which breast to offer next:

> It's just getting her used to it and once my milk kicks in a bit more as well (*laughs*) ... and another thing that worries me (*laughs*) is which breast I've fed her on, like remembering to swap over each time, so she gets a proper feed. I've been writing them down on a piece of paper ticking them off like (*laughs*), but like last night she'd only feed for like a couple of minutes on one and then she was on for like nearly an hour on the other, so ... like ... I was trying to, you know, balance it out like.
>
> (Millie, P43)

Previous experience constituted an important influence upon confidence in breastfeeding both in terms of 'producing' and 'delivering', with positive experiences increasing confidence and negative experiences having the potential to lower confidence depending upon how they were overcome. Louise (P14) related to her previous experience and feeling of lack of control:

> I get very hung up about things, like last time he didn't gain weight ... in the end the doctor said we'd better put him on the bottle. I was very stressed and I could have fed him all day and it wouldn't have filled him up. Once I had stopped the doctor said maybe I could give him a morning, midday and evening feed, but once I gave up, within a day and a half my milk had disappeared completely. I don't think he was getting anything and I think it was a combination of things, including a lack of control. This time I'm hoping that things will be different.
>
> (Louise, P14)

Women were aware that lack of previous experience contributed to them feeling less confident:

> I'm not very confident yet (*laughs*), cos I've read the books, I think I've read too many books, but I think you need practical experience which I haven't had, but I feel more confident than I did yesterday (*laughs*), but it's things like holding her which make me feel less confident. Like we haven't got any babies in the family, so it's quite hard ... But, I'll just keep trying. She is latching on but she doesn't seem to be getting very much. It's hard work, because she's not used to it and you're not used to it; you know it's a skill.
>
> (Selina, P48)

Women who had breastfed before tended to feel more relaxed and confident:

> With it being my second ... I'm more relaxed this time (*laughs*) ... The problem I had with my other little girl was that one of my nipples was inverted and

I used to find it was difficult to latch her on to it, because she actually had to suck at it to draw the nipple out, so that was a bit frustrating. But I'm aware of that – it seems easier with Louise, probably again, because of my confidence, she seems to be able to suck on it and get the nipple extended ... It's certainly easier the second time.

(Shirley, P57)

It is argued that women need to be prepared for the insecurity and uncertainty of breastfeeding with regards to quantification (Marchand and Morrow 1994; Mozingo *et al.* 2000). This preparation was not evident in the interactions I observed between midwives and mothers. Indeed, healthcare staff tended to employ a range of mechanistic assumptions related to breastfeeding, suggesting that they also saw breastfeeding primarily as a source of nutrition for feeding the baby's physical body with breast milk needing to be transferred effectively. Chloe (P50), whose baby had been born at thirty-seven weeks gestation, was undermined by the paediatrician's comments regarding her baby getting enough calories:

She doesn't seem to suck for very long then she gazes round the place, so I'm a bit uncertain as to whether she's actually getting enough milk, what's it called, colostrum. I got really concerned about it, so she had a cup feed yesterday. She took that down really quickly. That was at 4 o'clock yesterday afternoon, so I thought then, well I'm not giving her enough. I mean she hadn't really fed for about 12 hours. It was the paediatrician – she came round yesterday and it was shortly after that that she had a cup feed, because she said you need to make sure she's getting the calories from the milk and I thought, oh, I've got no way of knowing, you know.

(Chloe, P50)

In a number of interactions midwives emphasised that the baby was big in a way that appeared to link size with potential insufficiency of milk; for example:

*Virginia (MW20):*    Have you leaked any colostrum while you were pregnant?
*Sue (P29):*          Yeah
*Virginia:*           You have. Mmm; he's a big baby.

References to the baby's hunger were sometimes made; for example Hannah (P49) was holding her baby who had hiccups. Isabel (MW34) went past and said, 'Oooh ... what's the matter with you, are you hungry?'

Midwives tended to indicate ways in which women could see or know that they had breast milk; for example Felix (MW29) suggested that Selina (P48) look for signs of colostrum through expressing:

Felix:    Do you want to try expressing a little bit of milk onto your nipple?
*(Selina squeezes her nipple in a way that is unlikely to yield any colostrum.)*

*Selina:* *(on seeing that no milk is evident)* This is what I'm worried about, there's
   nothing there.
*Felix:* Not everyone can express colostrum ... so don't worry.

Having suggested that Selina expressed colostrum Felix then indicated that not
everyone could express colostrum, clearly giving mixed messages. As part of the
same dialogue, Felix emphasised progression to the next stage:

*Felix:* Are your breasts starting to feel any fuller?
*Selina:* They're a bit tender, but that's all.
*Felix:* You should start to feel a bit fuller by about tonight.
*Selina:* Tonight, oh.

Selina was very anxious about what the baby was getting. She was still not attaching her baby to the breast effectively. By the third day her breasts were still soft
and the baby had received a cup feed as he appeared to be dehydrated.

Women were repeatedly 'reassured' that things would be all right when their
milk came through. Damaris (MW18) came to see how Grace's baby was feeding
(she was first-day post-Caesarean section):

*Damaris (MW18):* Oh he's doing fine.
*Grace (P28):* There doesn't seem to be much there, he keeps coming off.
*Damaris:* You'll have colostrum which will usually see him through,
   then your milk will come in about the third day.

Here Damaris referred to colostrum as 'usually' seeing a baby through which
implicitly suggests that it may not. Second, she reiterates the linear fracturing of
procreative events and progression to the next stage referred to by Simonds
(2002) and discussed above. Midwives often 'reassured' women by emphasising
that what goes in necessarily comes out, a mechanistic expression typical of the
western conceptualisation of the body as machine (Helman 1994). However, as
seen above with Alison (P38), this led to insecurity if the expected output did not
occur on a particular day. The following interaction illustrates this issue:

*Chloe (P50):* I'm not sure she's feeding enough?
*Isabel (MW34):* Is she weeing and pooing?
*Chloe:* Yes.
*Isabel:* Well, if there isn't anything else going in there wouldn't be any-
   thing coming out.
*Chloe:* Oh.
*Isabel:* And she was suckling and gulping before so that shows you
   she's getting something.
*Chloe:* Oh.

| *Isabel:* | We'll leave it until she's a bit more alert and then we'll see how she's feeding. |
|---|---|
| *Chloe:* | All right. |

The ritual of weighing the baby while in hospital was testimony to the continued use of mechanistic ways of assessing output. The practice of weighing in hospital has been discontinued in some maternity units for healthy term babies. However, here the practice was still in evidence. The babies were weighed at birth on delivery suite and thereafter every other day, i.e. third, fifth, etc. Weighing was generally referred to as something that happens and was not discussed as a choice:

| *Kim (MW15):* | You know we'll be weighing tomorrow. We weigh on the third day. We'll weigh him tomorrow but you know he'll lose 10 per cent of his birth weight; breastfed babies do. Bottle fed babies don't because they're getting the full amount straight away. |
|---|---|
| *Barbara (P37):* | Oh, I didn't know that. |
| *Kim:* | Once your milk comes in he'll be more settled. |

Here Kim's language implied that breastfeeding would not provide the 'full amount' in the early days, linking it to a weight loss. The weighing ritual was generally conducted with little background discussion or explanation:

| *Holly (MW7):* | You know they lose up to 10 per cent of their weight? (As she lifted her on to the scales.) |
|---|---|
| *Vicky (P30):* | Do they? Oh. |
| *Holly:* | Six to eight. |
| *Vicky:* | Is that all right? |
| *Holly :* | I need to convert it over. *(Focused on the chart.)* Yeah, you're fine there. You can dress her now. |

Weighing appeared to increase some women's anxieties about their breast milk even though they were informed that up to 10 per cent weight loss was normal; for example:

> She's lost ten ounces, but ... er it's only 10 per cent of her original weight, so, she's allowed to lose that ... Um, I didn't like the fact that she lost weight ... Even though they said it was normal. It made me think, why's she lost weight, has she not been fed properly?
>
> (Carol, P31)

Midwives had mixed feelings about weighing, tending to do it because they were required to. However, some midwives clearly disliked the procedure:

I feel very negative about this weighing. I mean the scales we use ... you need the reflexes of a fighter pilot to get an accurate reading. Then, OK, if the reading is positive it reassures women, in fact they seem to ask for it, even if it is not offered. It's a number to go on. They've been conditioned to expect it. But what happens when the weight is down, mothers do a nose dive. Babies can be assessed without numbers. I think all midwives should have a month here without access to scales or weighing. It would make them use other means to assess a baby. They would have to watch the baby.

(Jenny, MW14)

Weighing may be seen as the ultimate way of monitoring and surveillance of an otherwise unpredictable process – breastfeeding. This has certainly been the case in the past when medicalisation of infant feeding reached its zenith (Balsamo *et al.* 1992; Vincent 1999). In this way weighing of the baby represents the continuing influence of authoritative medical knowledge and surveillance upon women's experiences of breastfeeding (Dykes and Williams 1999; Dykes 2002; Sachs 2005).

### Breastfeeding as labour

As illustrated, women expressed deep-seated doubts about their ability to 'produce' and 'deliver' their breast milk to their baby. In relation to women's ways of experiencing breastfeeding in hospital, I contend that this data represents an extension of Martin's (1987) industrial model applied to labouring women. Martin frames her analysis within Marxist notions of the people's alienation and separation from the product of their labour. In accordance with this model, she argues that the labouring woman is disconnected from her birth, seeing it as something that is managed and controlled by the system. To recap, Martin portrays labour as a production process with the woman as the labourer, her uterus as the machine, her baby as the product and the doctor as the factory supervisor or owner. Thus, she asserts, women come to see their bodies as defined by the implicit scientific metaphors that assume that, 'women's bodies are engaged in "production" with the separation this entails (given our conception of production) between labourer and labourer, labourer and product, labourer and labour, and manager and labourer' (194). The later empirical work of Davis-Floyd (1992, 1994) in the US yielded similar conclusions to Martin as a large number of women saw their bodies as vessels through which specific functions could be performed. They expressed open acceptance of the techno-medical aid on offer to supplement their body's activities. Davis-Floyd (1992) refers to these women as being conceptually fused with the technocratic model of birth.

In extending Martin's model to breastfeeding women on postnatal wards, breastfeeding becomes the production process, the woman is still the labourer and her breasts now replace the uterus as the key functional machines. Now breast milk becomes the product, with her baby assuming the role of consumer. If the breasts (machines) are in 'good working order' then they will 'produce' the right amount and quality of the 'product', breast milk. If they are used effectively by the labourer, then they will transfer the 'product' efficiently and effectively and in the correct amount to the 'consumer', the baby. However, given that the above processes are seen as prone to unreliability and failure, supervision is required. In the UK this role is largely designated to the midwife, who assumes the role of shop-floor supervisor. This series of mechanistic metaphors aids understanding regarding women's lack of confidence in their role as accountable producer. As Lupton (1996) states, the 'infant's body becomes a symbol of a mother's ability to feed and care for it well' (42). This well-being or otherwise is visible and open to surveillance and the mother subsequently exposes herself to blame.

This biomedical and mechanistic view of breastfeeding stands in stark contrast to the holistic conceptualisations in some non-westernised communities; for example parts of rural India. Here breastfeeding is seen more as a total mind–body experience, enhancing a knowing and love between mother and baby and transmitting emotions, cultural knowledge and moral character to the baby. If the mother has good thoughts during breastfeeding then her baby will grow up to be a good listener and a well-balanced person (Spiro 1994, 2006; Vincent 1999). It is interesting, however, to note that whatever the cultural beliefs about breast-feeding, the potential for blaming the mother is ever present (Spiro 1994, 2006; Jolly 1998; Vincent 1999).

In conclusion, the notion of 'supplying' relates to the discursive reduction of breast milk to a substance that is valued for its components (Van Esterik 1988; Blum 1993; Dettwyler 1995; Nadesan and Sotirin 1998) and to women's lived experiences of breastfeeding. Women appeared to conceptualise their bodies as vessels that were apart from them. There was a sense of alienation and separation from the product, breast milk. These dualistic understandings of bodies were rein-forced within the hospital setting through the mechanistic language of midwives. Women reflected their deep mistrust in the efficacy of their bodies and a profound lack of personal confidence, unless they had breastfed with some degree of felt success previously. When conceptualising their bodies in this way, as machines, the task was inevitably seen as demanding. In the next section I make a connec-tion between women's embodiment of the requirement to produce and deliver breast milk and their anxieties related to the experience of feeding their babies 'on demand'.

## Demanding

The concept of demand feeding appeared in western literature in the 1950s (Illingworth and Stone 1952) but did not become a firmly established concept until the 1980s. The concept came about with the recognition that if babies are given unlimited and untimed access to their mother's breast then they would be able to regulate their own calorific and nutritional requirements. This body of knowledge has grown over the last thirty years and is summarised by Woolridge

(1995). Demand feeding is associated with increased duration for which women breastfeed (Illingworth and Stone 1952; Slaven and Harvey 1981; Martines *et al.* 1989). The notion of demand feeding represents a dramatic reversal of the authoritative knowledges presented in the earlier decades of the twentieth century, in which scheduling of feeding was reified. Demand feeding is interchangeably referred to as baby-led feeding (Woolridge 1995; UNICEF 2001), although the principles underpinning the relationship are unchanged. The term 'demand' constitutes an industrial metaphor that links with the notion of the production line. The concept of the baby demanding a feed and indeed her/his demands being willingly met day and night is, however, antithetical to many of the beliefs around childcare which have developed since the Enlightenment.

In this chapter I highlight the ways in which demand feeding was experienced by women as breaching temporal and spatial boundaries, as constructed within UK culture. To assist in conceptualising the ways in which 'demand feeding' is perceived in a western culture, I return to the notion of linear and cyclical time. Spiro's (1994, 2006) research with Gujarati women was particularly illuminating in relation to cultural interpretations of time. She utilised an ethnographic approach to study the meaning of breastfeeding for Gujarati women living in Harrow, UK. Her findings illustrate that the women who had recently lived in rural communities in Gujarat had an agricultural, cyclical concept of time, related to the sun and the seasons rather than the clock. However, those who spent longer in a western culture developed a more linear concept of time, the extent of which related to the length of time in the latter community. She therefore illustrates that cyclical and linear time may be seen as poles, with women being positioned along a continuum between them. Spiro (1994, 2006) reports that for rural Gujarati women, time is rhythmical and seasonal with breastfeeding being part of the cycle of life. Childbirth and breastfeeding are seen as 'time out', a time of rest, with the mother's relationship with the baby being seen as a time of intimacy, mutuality, harmony and flexibility. This 'time out', which is common in many cultures around the world (Baumslag and Michels 1995; Vincent 1999), stands in total contrast to the experiences of some women in the UK.

Kahn (1989) refers to a form of time that relates to cyclical time, which she names 'maialogical time' (27). Using this neologism, she refers to the period during a woman's life when she bears children and lactates. She develops the word from the Greek word 'maia' which means to mother or nurse. This word maia originated from the Indo-European root 'ma' which derives from the notion of the child's cry for the breast. She chooses this word stem because it is free from male construction and second because it gives voice to the baby, 'from a maialogical perspective childbirth becomes the founding moment of the relation of self to other, grounded in the body, since both the *one being born* and the *one giving birth* are taken into account' (Kahn 1989: 27). Kahn contrasts the concept of maialogical time with linear time. The former embraces mutuality, interrelatedness, interaction and reciprocity. It relates to the relational self, that is a 'self essentially related to others in mind and body' (28). Linear time, she states, is:

inhabited by individuated western man who follows the linear trajectory of history, a trajectory considered to be healthy [...] its sociability is based upon the collective activity of 'autonomous' individuals frequently in competition with one another, or working for the benefit of someone else at the expense of the self.

(28)

Forman (1989) refers to Kahn's development of the notion of maiological time and argues that this concept of time would allow women as a collective to not only 'live *in* time' but to '*give* time' (7). This notion of being able, or indeed unable, to 'give time' arises throughout this book with regard to mothers and midwives.

It could be argued that many women in western industrialised cultures have become so programmed by linear (clock) time that they may be unable to enter or experience cyclical time (Kahn 1989; Adam 1992). However, it is important to avoid dualistic representations of living in and with time, suggesting that we can only engage with one form of time or another. Kahn (1989) indeed illustrates this with her own experiences of motherhood and feeding, which she argues allowed her to experience cyclical time in spite of living in linear time. She refers to her own experience of returning to work, where linear time predominated and contrasts it with her experience of cyclical time when breastfeeding her baby in the evening.

Kahn (1989) thus argues that women, through the experiences of pregnancy, birth and lactation, can potentially recover something of maiological time (29). However, she acknowledges that living in a culture where linear time dominates militates against this. Balsamo *et al.* (1992) likewise argue that breastfeeding is an experience that takes a person outside the industrial conception of time. However, as she argues, trying to negotiate the two types of time creates feelings of conflict for women. The data I present in this book, from women a decade later, when scheduling of feeds is no longer formally imposed, reflects similar tensions. I now discuss, in turn, two organising themes encompassed by the global theme of 'demanding': 'breaching temporal boundaries' and 'breaching bodily boundaries'.

### Breaching temporal boundaries

There is considerable ambiguity in relation to the notion of demand feeding, with contemporary breastfeeding texts referring to the need to allow a baby to feed without restriction. However, these texts often use biomedical language which remains distinctly time, transfer and measurement related, as illustrated in the following passage, in which I have italicised the words related to time:

It is advisable for numerous reasons to feed young infants whenever they indicate a desire to feed. When left to their own devices, infants feed for greatly *varying durations,* with *length* probably determined by the *rate and effectiveness* of milk transfer. Infants who are permitted to *regulate the frequency and duration* of their feeds *suckle more, gain weight more rapidly,* and *breastfeed for longer periods* than infants who are *restricted* in their *feeding patterns.*

(Saadeh and Akre 1996: 156)

Like the early biomedical literature on breastfeeding, the mother remains largely invisible here and any suggestion of mutuality and relationship is absent. The emphasis remains on efficient production and transfer of milk from mother to baby. These time-orientated constructions of demand feeding (Saadeh and Akre 1996) stand in stark contrast to the ways of feeding seen in cultures in which babies are carried on their mother's abdomens with constant access to the breast. As Palmer (1993) notes, to ask a mother in some cultures about the frequency of breastfeeds would be like asking her how often she scratches when she has an itch.

The ambiguities in the ways in which demand feeding may be described have the potential to create confusion for women. Women are still likely to have relatives and members of their communities who schedule-fed their babies, so the intergenerational conflict of ideas plays a role in increasing confusion. To complicate matters further, the authoritative knowledge pendulum is still in motion regarding these two approaches, with a resurgence of 'schedule' advocates; for example Ford (1999), who contests the notion of the baby being placed in control, with emphasis instead being placed on timing and discipline imposed by the parents.

The data from this study illustrates that women were indeed confused about demand feeding. They knew it involved a flexible approach, that is feeding the baby when s/he was hungry, but still often felt unsure about what this involved: 'I don't know whether I'm feeding him enough. How long should you feed when they are demanding?' (Helen, P35).

> I think in the night, it was more what I expected it to be, just sort of every four hours, but since eleven (now 5pm) it's just been constant ... I didn't expect that. It's all so contradictory, so many pros and cons ... You never truly know.
>
> (Barbara, P37)

While biomedical literature on demand feeding is extensive, there is little emphasis upon the ways in which women in a western culture interpret, experience and negotiate demand feeding their babies. In this study, demand feeding appeared to be central to women's experiences. The removal of culturally ingrained, linear temporal markers from a lived and embodied experience created considerable discord. The inherent irregularity, uncertainty and symbiotic assumptions underpinning demand feeding led to profound feelings of uncertainty. Women seemed to feel dislocated in time. Balsamo *et al.* (1992) refer to this 'social conditioning to order' in western communities, with unscheduled breastfeeding representing 'disorderliness' and being perceived as 'never-ending and exhausting' (74). The discord women experienced in relation to the variable and unpredictable nature of demand feeding is illustrated by Lesley:

> Basically he wasn't taking a lot and he was just taking little bits and I was winding him and seeing if he was interested, so I put him down and as soon as I put him down he was starting off again, but as soon as I put him back to my breast he was drinking again, so I was like ... what's going on? When I spoke to the midwife she said it was just down to my milk coming in, so ... I don't really know what I was expecting to be honest ... It's been a bit irregular and yesterday I don't know whether it was cos there was a lot of visitors around but he wasn't taking a lot. It was just little bits here and there and then I was winding him and putting him down and he wasn't settling and he was ... like ... he wanted more, so I was up till about 2 o'clock.
>
> (Lesley, P55)

This entire narrative is punctuated by time. Lesley's reference to her baby taking 'little bits' reflects what Helman (1992) refers to as the western linear assumption that 'every event or phenomenon will have both a beginning and an end' (37). In contrast, women felt confident if a baby stayed latched on to the breast for a period of time which they felt was acceptable; for example:

> I felt more confident once she'd actually latched on, and once she's there she tends to stay there. I think if she'd been mooching about and coming on and off all the time I think that would have made me really nervous.
>
> (Tracy, P44)

Women became anxious when there were changes in the 'pattern' of demand feeding: 'OK, she's been feeding every few hours, but she has not woken up since 5 so I'm feeling a bit like well, not so confident' (Megan, P53). Midwives used the language of demand feeding, but often appeared to have similar anxieties related to the uncertainty of breastfeeding; for example Sharlene saw demand feeding as an additional source of chaos:

> The wards are chaos. Medics and everyone else come and go all day. The midwives come and go and the babies feed whenever they want to ... When I fed mine we had a routine and it fitted in with my life – I could go to the supermarket and do some shopping. I was talking to someone the other day and she demand fed for a year and the baby just took over her life. Babies snacking all the time don't fit in with our culture and I think that's why women are giving up. It's difficult to sustain with current lifestyles.
>
> (Sharlene, MW6)

One of the midwives highlighted some of the tensions for midwives and other women related to their personal attitudes on demand feeding:

> I think midwives tend to be guided by what worked for them, no matter how many courses you go on, you tend to do what works for you. I think demand feeding is one of the slowest items of all. Mothers come in with this idea of four hourly feeds, they have that expectation and they're concerned if the baby goes longer and they're concerned if they go more frequently. I think that's part of the tension around breastfeeding; they have this expectation of three or four hourly, timetabled feeding and when a baby is feeding virtually continuously or on and off for long, long periods they think there's something wrong, that they've not got enough milk or the baby is excessively hungry.
>
> (Jenny, MW14)

Most of the women including the midwives spoke in ways that indicated a strong orientation towards the clock and a preoccupation with schedules, times and routines. As stated, the deep embeddedness of linear time in western bodies is in total contradiction to the concept of demand feeding. In spite of women referring to themselves as carrying out demand feeding, they were intensely preoccupied with frequencies and durations of feeds, referring to these with meticulous reference to the clock:

> Well, she had a proper feed just before visiting hours, like ... and then another feed just after visiting hours, like for about forty-five minutes and she was sucking really hard and that was on each breast and then about twelve o'clock from then on till half five she was like feeding and then sleeping and waking up and having more and that. Then they took her out then she had about a thirty-minute one at quarter to seven and after that she went to sleep until about ten o'clock.
>
> (Millie, P43)

The reference to a 'proper feed' by Millie appears to relate to women seeing breastfeeding as primarily a source of nutrition and therefore their expectations that babies would take a 'proper meal' of breast milk. As stated above, it is again reflective of the western linear assumption related to beginnings and ends (Helman 1992).

Midwives paid lip-service to the notion of demand feeding but in their language tended to give mixed messages by requesting fairly detailed information about the baby's frequency and duration of suckling; for example:

*Veronica* (P27):    He's feeding all the time.
*Damaris (MW18):*    He seems content at the moment. What time did he last feed?
*Veronica:*    An hour ago.
*Damaris:*    And what about previous to that?
*Veronica:*    A couple of hours before that.

| | |
|---|---|
| *Damaris:* | How long did he feed for? |
| *Veronica:* | Oh about half an hour or so. |

Damaris's preoccupation with frequency and duration of feeds reflects the common assumption that these measures can be equated with quantity of milk taken. While this assumption is fraught with problems in terms of physiological understandings (Woolridge 1995), it is understandable in relation to western associations between time and quantity. As Adam (1992) states, 'Clock time, the organizational frame and structure of industrial production is governed by the non-temporal principle of invariant repetition. Objectified and reified it is related to as a quantity' (160).

The adherence to the philosophy of measurement of feed frequencies and durations was at its most striking in paediatric advice issued in case notes, as described by Jenny (MW14). She referred to the philosophy of demand feeding as being totally antithetical to paediatricians' ways of knowing and working, representing them as being at the extreme end of a range of views related to flexibility versus routines for breastfeeding:

> Demand feeding ... it's an endless source of tension with paediatricians. For a normal baby, the paediatricians have this idea of regular feeds and they frequently write it on the charts when called to delivery for something like meconium liquor or low Apgar. Even when resuscitation hasn't been needed or has been successful, they'll put 'plan', to ward with mother, monitor temperature, four hourly temps, three hourly feeds, early feeding. It's like a mantra really, and you've got a strong, healthy normal baby who doesn't need any particular regime at all. You know the paediatric chart with the tick list, when the paediatrician has been at delivery, you'll see that on almost every one. It's the beginning of pathologising.
>
> (Jenny, MW14)

This illustrates the point made by Thomas (1992) that 'time provides not only ways of describing the distribution of events but also a basis for interpretations and explanations' (65).

During the analysis I became increasingly aware of the mothers' expectations of a 'good baby', that is one that limits his/her demands. This was part of women's project to produce the perfect adult for their own society. This project commenced before or during pregnancy, to include decisions around feeding method, but it continued following the birth. The requirement upon mothers to tame their baby and prepare her/him for the requirements of and scrutiny by the society of that time were discussed in Chapter 2, with particular reference to the historical analysis by Beekman (1977) of child-rearing practices. Whichever philosophy of parenting and infant feeding that women adopt in a given western society, they were and are still expected to civilise their baby (Lupton 1996; Schmied 1998; Meyer and de Oliveira 2003). As Lupton (1996) states, 'mothers domesticate children, propelling them from the creature of pure instinct and uncontrolled wildness of infancy into the civility and self-regulation of adulthood' (39). Food and eating have constituted a key route to achieving this civility throughout recorded history (Fildes 1986; Maher 1992a, 1992b; Vincent 1999).

The project of producing a future citizen for our society is an extremely complex and culturally mediated endeavour. In the data that I have presented so far, and the data I move on to include, I illustrate that mothers and midwives are still preoccupied to varying degrees with the baby being able to develop routines, be 'good', passive and docile. This involved the baby not being too demanding, sleeping for acceptable periods and not playing at the breast. This expectation appeared to run alongside the desire that the baby would be capable of early independence and even separation, that is willing to take a dummy, sleep in the cot and able to engage in self-amusement. The following interview with Millie highlights some of these issues:

> She was just crying for nothing really ... She just wanted to be cuddled, but she'd been cuddled all night ... and I was asking this morning, like, do you think I should just leave her in the cot and let her just cry and try to rock her to sleep or take her out and feed her and she [the midwife] said I don't think she needs a feed now, she's just doing it to get into bed with you ... just feed her and then put her down and I did but she wouldn't settle properly, so I had to get her up. I think I should be able to cope when she gets into a routine and especially once I get home. I'll be able to sleep better in my own bed ... you know. What's worrying me is the fact that she is up in the night and it is demand feeding. If she wants to feed she will cry until she gets fed, you know, whether I'm ready to feed her or not ... and you can't tell, you know, as much ... whether she's had enough or is she awake because she's awake or does she want feeding or ... because she will latch on and sometimes she just falls asleep and starts playing and I think that's when she just wants to play. She doesn't want feeding and I mean that worries me a little bit, because obviously it's keeping me awake all night.
>
> (Millie, P43)

The midwife clearly reinforced the sense that the baby was simply 'playing up' in her suggestion that the baby was trying to get into her mother's bed and Millie was concerned that this night-time behaviour would be a major inconvenience by keeping her awake. Women also referred to having or desiring a 'good baby':

> I've kept an open mind if it didn't work ... like I know people who have breast fed ... um ... you know for ages ... you know ... with both their children ... and I know another couple of people who just couldn't get the hang of it and just turned to bottles straight away ... and their babies have been absolutely fine ... there's nothing ... you know ... they slept and they were

good babies ... so I've kept an open mind so that I wouldn't be disappointed ... if he needs the bottle.

(Sophie, P61)

Tracy saw good behaviour as not messing around:

Yesterday, I felt a bit (*negative gesture*) ... because she wasn't feeding, but then as soon as she started feeding in the night, I felt OK. She either feeds or she doesn't, she's quite good; she won't just sort of mess with it all the time.

(Tracy, P44)

It seems that women expected their babies to fit certain activities into specific, bounded sections of time, as Helman (1992) states, 'the clock – as a crucial organising principle in industrial society – symbolizes control, conformity and co-operation in social and economic life' (43). As stated, women appeared to expect passivity and docility in their baby, yet desired steady and visible progress towards independence. The data illustrates women's dissonance related to competing agendas of being a flexible, child-centred responsive parent and training the baby to conform to societal norms. This discord strongly resonates with the findings of Schmied (1998). It could be argued that passive dependence on consumables, yet independence from the mother, is best achieved through bottle feeding a baby with infant formula. Van Esterik (1995) highlights the fundamental difference between breast and bottle feeding, in that with the former, the baby, if permitted to engage in demand feeding, can actively control the way in which s/he drinks milk. The bottle-fed infant, she argues, is passive, controlled by others, and becomes a dependent consumer from birth (161).

Vincent (1999) refers to the emphasis in the earlier decades of the twentieth century upon infants needing to be disciplined through an 'external schedule to accustom their nervous systems to certain types of food, rest and play' (53). This was seen to prepare the infant for a scheduled life and the constraints of the clock that would be a major feature of their life as adults. However, she argues that by the 1960s the timetable was not simply seen as an external means of imposing discipline. Rather it came to be seen as an innate characteristic of the child. She states:

The clock has moved from the realm of culture as perceived in science, training and discipline to that of nature and organic processes. It has moved from outside to inside the human body [...]. The clock having been internalised is now thought to be inherent in human behaviour. Schedules are considered necessary for many activities such as work, sports, leisure, family life and have become a standard for judging competence, adequacy and normality. Thus the expectation that babies will conform to a feeding timetable, even though it may derive from their internal needs, is a reflection of a general cultural expectation that all behaviour is governed by schedules. The clock is at the core of many cultural themes and it is not surprising that it is still considered to be a fundamental element of infant feeding, even though the way it is described has changed.

(Vincent 1999: 54)

As discussed earlier, the clock has indeed become innate through its effects upon physiological processes (Helman 1992). However, this social conditioning to clock time could hardly be expected to be present in a baby only one or two days old. Women in this study did, however, appear to have the expectation that even if demand feeding was practised the baby should and would, after a short time, display her/his innate programming to get into a routine. Sophie anxiously awaited the development of a routine, giving the impression that if this did not happen soon she would reconsider her feeding options:

He's slept and settled but it's my first day and sometimes they don't feed as much on the first day do they, so ... I'll see how I go on through tonight and tomorrow and um ... see if he gets in a routine ... I think if he was in a routine ... I could feed him for 20 minutes/half and hour and then three hours later ... four hours later he'd take it again.

(Sophie, P61)

Kate clearly saw her baby as having moved positively in the direction of establishing a routine:

She seems to be getting into a bit more of a routine and at the last feed she didn't have as long on. She's had a bath this morning too at 08.15. Then she fed at nine and she's just fed now, for about twenty or thirty minutes.

(Kate, P39)

Smale (1996) highlighted a similar expectation in some of her clients, 'that a period of total unpredictability would resolve into a set regime' (236). Thus demand feeding tends to be seen as a transient phase that, in time, will resolve to a conformity to external and indeed internal clock time. The emphasis (above) upon babies behaving and *conforming* to clock time is in stark contrast to research around babies *taking time*. The notion of babies taking time is referred to in the feminist literature; for example Kahn (1989) highlights that babies live in maialogical time illustrating our fundamental sociability from birth. She refers to babies' innate abilities and tendencies that are particularly evident following an unimpeded birth. For example, the baby actively, indeed interactively, displays sociable gestures and makes her/his way to the mother's breast and suckles; this then encourages placental separation. The baby, therefore, initiates her/his realignment to her/his mother. Kahn (1989) argues that maialogical time is slow, enabling babies to display sociability and illustrate their 'integration into the organic cycle of life' (29). She refers to the 'baby's embeddedness in organic or cyclical time, which knows nothing of the clock' (22). Hannah, who had several children, illustrated the notion of babies being given time to take their time:

> I'd say for everybody to just bear with it, because a lot of people want to breastfeed, but because the baby won't take off them they tend to get upset as well. I think that that should be put on leaflets and stuff, because it's very frustrating if you want to do something, but your baby won't do it. They need to point out that it's not just your baby that's like that, and that if your baby doesn't take to it straight away it's not that it's discontented with you but it's just taking time ... just put the baby in the nighty and lie with them at night or when they're cuddling them and they will eventually mooch.
>
> (Hannah, P49)

However, Hannah's emphasis upon babies 'taking their time' in contrast to babies 'taking up time', was rarely referred to by mothers or midwives. It seems that an explanation around this principle might well alleviate considerable anxiety in women. If women understood the concept of maialogical time they might feel less pressured about their babies' need for time with them. However, the drive to establish routines in childcare and to return to a 'normal' life as quickly as possible are in tension with this notion of maialogical time. There was a sense in the data which resonates with that of others (Schmied 1998; Mahon-Daly and Andrews 2002) that women felt their lives were 'on hold' (Schmied 1998: 292). While this is the predominant feeling, breastfeeding will continue to be seen as short term, marginal and disruptive. I now turn to another way in which women felt that breastfeeding encroached on their boundaries, though space rather than time.

### Breaching bodily boundaries

The second organising theme underpinning 'demanding' was 'breaching bodily boundaries'. Women tended to express discord in relation to the erratic disruption to spatial bodily boundaries caused by demand feeding. Breastfeeding as a lived, embodied experience constituted an intermittent disrupting of their bodily boundaries with previously invisible spatial norms being violated. Women's concerns appeared to be closely linked to a partial fear of intensive mothering and an accompanying desire to place control and distance within the feeding and mothering encounter. These concerns were also reported by Schmied (1998) in her Australian study, although she focused upon the ongoing experience of breastfeeding for women, not on the hospital period. She reported that for some women, some of the time, breastfeeding with its commitment to intensive mothering was experienced as a draining, disconnected and disruptive experience (Schmied 1998; Schmied and Barclay 1999).

The sense of disruption to spatial boundaries that women expressed while in hospital illustrated the way in which the breastfeeding experience contrasts with the predominant ontological position of western culture which centres around the separate, self-sufficient, independent, rational self or individual (Mauthner and Doucet 1998: 125). Shildrick (1997) refers to the leakiness of women's bodies breaching socially prescribed boundaries: 'those differences – mind/body, self/other, inner/outer – which should remain clear and distinct are threatened by loss of definition, or by dissolution' (17). In relation to inner and outer, women's bodies are contrasted with the 'self-contained and self-containing men', being seen as leaky and uncontained (34). In relation to self and other, Shildrick (1997) states:

> The indeterminacy of body boundaries challenges that most fundamental dichotomy between self and other, unsettling ontological certainty and threatening to undermine the basis on which the knowing self establishes control [...]. The capacity to be simultaneously both self and other in pregnancy, which is the potential of every woman, is the paradigm case of breached boundaries.
>
> (35)

When women have a new baby and begin to breastfeed, the breaching of boundaries is intensified as they undertake a profoundly new bodily experience. Their body's boundaries are now accessed with increasing unpredictability by another, further blurring the distinctions between self and other. Their breast milk comes from within and is manifest without through a part of their body that is constructed as both maternal and sexual in nature. Not only does the woman now need to come to terms with her unboundedness in relation to the baby, but she also has a re-negotiation of private and public space. She now shares her private space with her baby and in hospital she and her baby are also together in a very public place. This adds further blurring to the woman's sense of self in relation to others. Lupton (1996) refers to the ways in which breastfeeding breaches the boundaries between other and self:

> Just as the fetus/mother is a highly ambiguous category of subjectivity, there is a liminal stage between the mother's body and the infant's body, in which the milk acts as the connection; the milk is generated by the mother, taken in by the infant held close to the breast and becomes part of the infant's body. This liminality arouses anxieties around the defining of boundaries between self/other and nature/culture.
>
> (45)

Van Esterik (1994) likewise refers to experience of 'other as self – that makes breastfeeding both a powerful transforming experience for some and a terrifying loss of personal autonomy for others (or both at the same time)' (S47). Schmied (1998) also refers to breastfeeding as challenging dualistic boundaries between mind–body, nature–culture, inside–outside and motherhood–sexuality. Indeed, it could be argued that it is the ultimate form of breaching boundaries, hence its dangerous possibilities (Foucault 1981).

The most common way in which women expressed discord around breaching of spatial boundaries centred around use of their breasts as 'dummies':

I'm worried about using the nipple as a comforter, and I know you've got to demand feed, but, I don't want her to be permanently on (*laughs*) ... That's why I want to wean her off it before I go back to work, because obviously I'm going back, not quite full time, but thirty hours a week, so it'll be more difficult to sort of demand feed and what have you through the night.

(Nadine, P60)

Nadine's reference to the nipple, and weaning her off it, further illustrates women's objectification and conceptual detachment from their breasts. Women tended to describe sucking for comfort or using them as a dummy as unacceptable: 'He wants to have something in his mouth all the time' (Julie, P9); 'I think he was using it as a dummy last night, he seemed to be feeding for ages, like just wanting it next to his mouth' (Sarah, P10).

Barbara reiterated these concerns and emphasised that it should not become a 'habit', preferring that he learn to 'relax in the cot':

I mean feeding is a last resort, but I don't want it to become like a dummy, just a comfort thing. Um, I don't mind, but I'm a bit concerned because once he's on he just falls asleep. He doesn't actually take anything, as I was saying it's just a comfort thing ... Um, I don't want him just on me for no reason (*laughs*) ... I'm a bit don't know what to do really ... I am just concerned that it's going to be a habit, that I don't want to ... I really don't want it to be a habit where he's needed this much. I mean comfort wise I want him to relax in the cot rather than this.

(Barbara, P37)

Some women felt that by wanting to remain at the breast, the baby was engaging in unnecessary dependency upon them, 'I'm not always sure when she's had enough. She's quite content to hold my nipple, so it's knowing when to put her down ... like she's depending on me' (Jane, P12); 'She's needing it all the time, you know, I can't get away from the bed' (Stella, P46).

Midwives tended to reinforce the view that babies were using their mother's breast as a dummy, 'don't let him use you as a dummy'(Francesca, MW28); 'Is he using you for comfort?' (Kim, MW15). One of the midwives emphasised that babies suck for nurture as well as nutrition, although it was worded rather as an either/or scenario, 'they suck for nutrition, but sometimes they suck for comfort as well' (Sandy, MW30).

The interesting reversal from dummies replacing breasts, to breasts replacing dummies, highlights the strength of the pacifier as a cultural norm along with bottles and related paraphernalia in the west. This cultural reversal is characteristic of the bottle-feeding culture (Auerbach 1995; Wiessinger 1995, 1996). Indeed, as Weissinger (1996) argues, the cultural reversal has entered the language used in both professional and lay literature and spoken language so that bottle feeding and associated activities such as dummy usage are represented as the norm. Breastfeeding then becomes the activity to which we attribute difference.

Women felt that breastfeeding became particularly demanding when their bodily boundaries were actually broken, through the experience of sore nipples. The experience of nipple pain when breastfeeding is widely reported (Bowes and Domokos 1998; Schmied 1998; Schmied and Barclay 1999; Mozingo *et al.* 2000; Hamlyn *et al.* 2002; Woods *et al.* 2002). It is usually associated with ineffective attachment of the baby to the mother's breast (Woolridge 1986b) and may contribute to a disrupted, disconnected and distorted experience of breastfeeding for women (Schmied 1998; Schmied and Barclay 1999). It also contributes to dissonance with regard to expectation and reality (Bowes and Domokos 1998) and is the main reason for women in the UK discontinuing breastfeeding during the first week following their baby's birth (Hamlyn *et al.* 2002).

Of the sixty-one women I observed and spoke with, just over a third referred to their painful nipples, indicating that they were experiencing difficulties with effective attachment. Nipple pain in itself caused women to wonder whether they could continue. 'My nipple ... the pain is like ... it's debatable whether to carry on or not; they're starting to get really sore' (Megan; P53). Veronica changed to bottle feeding on her second night on the postnatal ward:

> It made me very, very sore. It just got progressively worse and worse, um last night, he was just constantly on the breast, sucking all the time. So I decided I'd had enough. It was a bit emotional. Um, so we've gone on to the bottle although it might not be for good. We'll have to see how it goes, after a few days, maybe ...
>
> (Veronica, P27)

Sadly, this scenario could have been avoided, in that sore nipples, such as experienced by Veronica, strongly suggest ineffective attachment of the baby to her/his mother's breast. The latter is commonly associated with an unsatisfied baby who may therefore want to breastfeed more frequently than s/he might otherwise, if s/he were able to feed effectively (Woolridge 1995). This was the basis upon which women used to be advised to restrict the duration and frequency of feeds when understanding regarding effective attachment of a baby to the mother's breast was minimal (Fisher 1985).

The support midwives provided for women with regard to nipple soreness was largely inadequate. This related in part to the many other calls upon their 'time' and partly to a lack of knowledge regarding effective attachment. Commonly, when women commented on soreness, midwives would indicate that the attachment/latch needed checking. However, they usually said they would come back and check it, but invariably did not. When they did 'check' the latch this often involved a transient glance and then they rushed off again. Often it was clear to me that the attachment and feeding dynamic was far from effective. There were only a few occasions when midwives sat and observed a feed.

Midwives did not appear to facilitate women in understanding how and why effective attachment would support breastfeeding. Carol was regularly 'checked' to see if she was doing it 'right', but she appeared to be none the wiser about what constituted effective attachment.

| | |
|---|---|
| *Carol (P31):* | Well, it's been really, really sore. I've been really sore and she was just wanting it more and more often. She was like feeding for an hour and she wanted it every half hour ... I've seen the midwife this morning and she's given me some Lansinoh cream (*shows me*). |
| *F:* | So how do your nipples feel now? |
| *Carol:* | Well, the cream has soothed them a bit, but they are cracked. |
| *F:* | So has anybody shown you how to attach the baby? |
| *Carol:* | Yeah, they've all checked and they said I have been doing it right ... if it doesn't get better in the next day, I don't think I'll be able to carry on, because I'm like that all the time (*grimaces*) when I'm feeding her and it's starting to make me feel ... put off feeding when it's like that ... it's just the pain. I do want to carry on, it's just overcoming the pain (*laughs*). |

Demand feeding and, by implication, using the mother as a 'dummy', was connected with nipple soreness by some midwives. Kim approached Barbara and took a quick glance at her breastfeeding, whilst stating:

| | |
|---|---|
| *Kim (MW15):* | Feeding again? |
| *Barbara (P37):* | I don't know if he's feeding really? |
| *Kim:* | Is he stopping and starting? |
| *Barbara:* | Yes. |
| *Kim:* | I'll come back in about half an hour and see how he's getting on. You're going to get sore otherwise aren't you? |

Again, this connection between length of feeding and nipple soreness may well have related to ineffective attachment, as from my own observation, the baby did not appear to be attaching effectively to the mother's breast.

Midwives commonly exhorted women to persevere through the pain:

> My nipples are very sore ... I just keep going, it makes your toes curl (*laughs*). One's better than the other you see which is quite common apparently ... The midwife just said to keep persevering, um ... they will get better ... As my milk comes through, he'll probably not ... you know guzzle, chomp quite as much you know ... Suck quite as hard sort of thing.
>
> (Corinne, P41)

While other researchers who apply a sociological perspective to breastfeeding identify the disruptive nature of sore nipples (Bowes and Domokos 1998; Schmied 1998; Schmied and Barclay 1999; Mozingo *et al.* 2000), they do not elaborate on the potential for changing the nature of the relationship and women's feelings about breastfeeding, through providing support with effective attachment. Such a focus moves research onto the edges of the 'breastfeeding management' domain which is carefully avoided as it stands in contradiction to the epistemological assumptions underpinning sociological research. However, given the current understandings of the relationships between ineffective attachment and sore nipples (Woolridge 1986b), this is an area which requires highlighting, as effective support from midwives has the potential to enhance women's lived experiences of breastfeeding.

Feelings of exhaustion and fatigue also contributed to women feeling that their boundaries were disrupted. Fatigue is recognised as a part of the postnatal experience of women, particularly manifesting in the first few days following the birth (Ball 1994; Cuttini *et al.* 1995; Rice *et al.* 1999; Rice 2000; McQueen and Mander 2003). It is a feature and challenge of early motherhood (Flagler 1990; Ball 1994; Barclay *et al.* 1997; Larkin and Butler 2000) and tends to be connected by women with breastfeeding (Vogel and Mitchell 1998; Mozingo *et al.* 2000; Hauck *et al.* 2002).

The combination of a baby feeding 'all the time' and the mother feeling that she didn't have enough time to sleep increased the feelings that breastfeeding was demanding. The fatigue tended to be connected by women to what they felt was prolonged or frequent feeding:

> Well, she had two very long goes at feeding overnight, like for an hour or so each and then she needs winding for about forty minutes, so I didn't get much sleep really.
>
> (Megan, P53)

Women struggled to relax at night due to the busy nature of the wards. The second night seemed to be particularly difficult for mothers. They had often been awake through the first night in a state of excitement and then by night two the fatigue was becoming intense. This existing tiredness was compounded by frequent feeding and sleeplessness on the postnatal ward: 'I can't keep this up for long, because he was born in the night so I didn't get any sleep that night. I need some sleep' (Barbara, P37 – third morning).

### Surreal moments

It was very striking that the notion of breastfeeding being demanding in various ways was reported by almost all of the participants I interviewed, although this is not to say that this was always construed negatively. There were several women who described breastfeeding as a positive embodied experience, even at this early stage, and this overrode some of the challenges.

Women sometimes reflected back to their experience of skin-to-skin contact with their baby after the birth, 'I held her close, next to my skin and I cried my eyes out. I couldn't believe that she came from my own body, I was awake all night. So excited you know' (Usha, P36).

> It's a very surreal moment ... I thought actually before oh, I'd like him cleaned up and you know wrapped up, and (*laughs*) ... No it was straight on and it was just wonderful ... then afterwards we were left with him and he was on my breast straight away then it was just the three of us. I'd thoroughly recommend it, you know, from being somebody who thought it would be nicer if we were all cleaned up. You don't care, and it's um, you know he was obviously all covered in blood and quite blue and not looking very babyish at that point, but it doesn't matter somehow; it's just a wonderful thing.
>
> (Alison, P38)

Alison described how this positive experience overrode her sense of 'orderliness' and 'cleanliness'. Some women referred to their first experience of breastfeeding as special, 'Um, dead special, really good ... I feel like closer to her' (Chris, P32); 'It was making me cry (*laughs*), not painful ... just because I was happy ... yeah' (Millie, P43).

Women also talked about special moments with their baby during their ongoing breastfeeding experience, 'I think it's such a nice moment to have with your baby' (Alison, P38); 'Well it's relaxing and you feel like you're bonding ... like you can cuddle and stare at the baby you know' (Sarah, P10); 'It's been lovely, he's really taken to it so far. I like the fact that I'm giving the feed not just sticking a bottle in his mouth. It's lovely' (Julie, P9).

Some women who had experienced ambivalence felt very differently as a result of breastfeeding and closeness with their baby. This gave them the desire to carry on: 'Now she's with me and breastfeeding I can feel the bonding and I have become convinced that I want to breastfeed' (Gemma, P5); 'It feels really natural. It wasn't what I expected, it's the strong bond ... It's nice actually, it just feels so right, so natural. I didn't think it would feel like this' (Jo, P45).

Denise emphasised a harmony between herself and her baby that made her desire to breastfeed entirely, 'I like the feeling that you are together – the feeling that he's accepted you really. I would like to try and breastfeed entirely now' (Denise, P4). This harmony, synchrony and mutuality was rarely mentioned at this early stage of breastfeeding, but is reported in relation to the ongoing relationship of breastfeeding for some women (Hewat and Ellis 1984; Bottorff 1990; Wrigley and Hutchinson 1990; Leff *et al.* 1994; Schmied and Barclay 1999).

Positive feelings were sometimes linked to feelings that the baby 'could do it'; 'It feels brilliant ... it feels nice that she can do it (Millie, P43). They also related to positive interpretations of the baby's temperament, known to contribute to a longer duration of breastfeeding (Leff *et al.* 1994; Vandiver 1997):

She took to it so quickly, really in the first few days ... I know she had a paddy last night, but she made it easy for me to feed, cos she was very easy, she was there, yes, she was easy ... I think if I'd have had a more difficult baby but she just latched on dead quickly; in some ways it's like I've been shown what to do, but she showed me, she's just been waiting to get on me and she's done the rest really. So she's made it easier for me.

(Vicky, P30)

Part of this interpretation of temperament may relate to whether the mother is attaching and feeding her baby effectively, which will influence the baby's behaviour and responses to her. The reference to 'special moments' by women illustrates that even at this early stage a few women had positive embodied experiences that had the potential to change the nature and course of their breastfeeding experience. However, sadly, some developed sore nipples which changed the nature of the experience to a negative one during the first few days of breastfeeding. This potential for fluctuation between positive and negative interpretations of the breastfeeding experience is described by Schmied and Barclay (1999).

I now focus upon ways in which women negotiated the temporal and spatial uncertainty inherent in breastfeeding, their felt imperative to return to paid employment and their lack of trust in their ability to breastfeed.

## Gaining control – maintaining boundaries

I have focused on anxieties experienced by women in relation to providing, producing and delivering their breast milk to the baby. I have also illuminated the ways in which women experienced dissonance related to the inherent uncertainty of demand feeding and the blurring of boundaries between themselves and their babies. I now focus upon the ways in which women coped, and planned to cope with, the inherent tensions related to the embodied disorderliness of breastfeeding and concerns about how they would return to and manage their busy 'normal' lives once home and their return to 'productive' employment.

In a society in which productivity, in the industrial sense, is super-valued and with lives structured around daily routines, breastfeeding women are faced with multiple contradictions. Their bodily rhythms and flows and the maialogical time of their babies contrast with the socially dominant form of time, linear time. Kahn (1989) summarises this dilemma as she refers to western industrial societies where women are subjected to an institution of motherhood in which they are expected to mother within a social system dominated by linear time. This expectation upon women centres upon a form of time which is 'extremely inhospitable to the slower tempo of children' in a culture in which there is little support for women who are still asked to put in most of the 'time' in the care of the young (28).

Women are now increasingly engaged in two forms of production, reproductive and industrial, and this creates specific pressures upon them (Galtry 1997a,

1997b, 1997c, 2000). One of these pressures centres upon conflicting notions of temporality. Balsamo *et al.* (1992) eloquently summarise the tensions between the 'natural' time of women's inherent bodily rhythms, flows and fluctuations and 'production' or 'social' time:

> Milk comes as the contractions of labour come and then the child and before them all, menstruation, breaking into patterns of social time. They have rhythms of their own, linked to the relationship of the woman to her physical and social background. They constitute a disturbance to the organisation of labour. And thus 'natural individual time' and the 'social time' of production come into conflict through the body of the woman. This conflict is even more dramatic today because production times have been accelerated with respect to 'natural' time, but also because women are becoming more and more integrated into the world of production and its forms of knowledge and are ever more dominated by it.
>
> (85)

The notion of the production line with its inherent super-valuation of speed, efficiency and productivity was central to women's concerns in my study. If time is seen as linear and related to efficiency and productivity in the industrial sense, then women will see breastfeeding as time-consuming and potentially time-wasting. This links with what Adam (1992) refers to as a notion of time as a quantifiable and finite resource with 'time running on and out' (162). She asserts that this conceptualisation is exclusive to a clock-time understanding of the world in total contrast to the notion of 'becoming' (163).

The fear of using up too much time was reflected in women's concerns related to the time between feeds and the time their babies slept for. Women's anxieties about the disordered and wasted time inherent in breastfeeding and the pressure upon them to get their bodies out into society and to engage with production as paid employees were evident within the first one to three days of their new mothering experiences. I was not expecting this finding in a hospital-based study when women had only just birthed. As a consequence of women's concerns, they endeavoured to place controls upon the timing and time taken in the act of breastfeeding. This conflict between women taking time out with their babies and resuming a 'normal' life to include getting back to work was ever present. There is now an entire service industry that separates out the supply function of the mother from the demands of the baby. Mothers can now express breast milk or give formula milk that may be issued to the baby by someone else, somewhere else. The baby's needs for nurture may be satisfied with a dummy rather than the breast. Meanwhile, the woman can restore her figure, put on her suit or jeans and stride out into the workplace in order to resume efficient productivity.

A glance at breast-pump advertisements in breastfeeding journals illustrates this philosophy perfectly as the well-dressed, slim woman may be seen marching off into the distance with breast pump in a smart compact briefcase. No doubt the case could also contain breast pads to prevent any sign of uncontrolled bodily flu-ids becoming evident. The baby is strikingly absent. Blum (1999) refers to the breast-milk feeding philosophy that has grown recently in the US:

> the breastfeeding-wage-earning supermom, who is, paradoxically, free from any embodied constraints or wants. She is treated and treats herself as nearly body-less, and can be endlessly self-disciplining [...]. Today's supermom gets medical approval to carry her breast pump to work, and, through her milk, to maintain her claim to exclusive, class enhancing motherhood.
>
> (183)

The marketing of the bottle, breast-milk substitutes and breastfeeding aids, dis-cussed in the background, is designed to target this 'modern' mother (Palmer 1993; Baumslag and Michels 1995; Sokol 1997), who is portrayed as confident in the work place, but paradoxically has little trust in her own body.

### Paradoxes of control

In this study, gaining and regaining control appeared to be very important to women. The concept of control relates not only to power and *being* controlled but also to individuals' desires and needs to feel *in control* of their lives and circum-stances in an endeavour to maintain predictability. Hastrup (1995) argues that in western cultures, control involves disengaging from our material selves, control-ling our bodily sources of error and making rational, instrumental decisions.

A paradox of control in the context of breastfeeding is that, like labour and childbirth, the process is at its most effective as an embodied experience when it involves relaxation and going with the 'flow', rather than trying to control it in an instrumental, goal-centred way (Odent 1992; Britton 1997). As Anderson (2000) states, 'letting go' occurs on a psychological level that allows the physical body to take control. Thus the woman still retains her sense of 'control', because she 'is the body that is in control' (96). The physiological connections are clear, in that in both labour and breastfeeding, release of the hormone oxytocin is hampered by adrenaline and noradrenaline, two hormones associated with stress (Odent 1992; Ueda *et al.* 1994; Nissen *et al.* 1998).

In spite of the physiological basis, this concept of 'letting go' directly contra-dicts the valued western concept of individuals exerting rational and instrumental control over their lives and bodies (Britton 1997). It also contra-venes the philosophy of western medicine with its profound fear of chaos and uncertainty in relation to the body and bodily processes and its consequent focus on controlling the body (Davis-Floyd 1994; Lupton 1994). This is partic-ularly relevant in relation to breastfeeding as a bodily secretion which brings with it all the fears of disorderly losses from the body as they leak, seep, gush, flow and surge (Foucault 1981; Martin 1987; Lupton 1994; Shildrick 1997; Bramwell 2001).

Women in this study were endeavouring to cope with and control three dimensions of temporality: the past, the present and the future. They were recovering and re-orientating from their labour and birthing experience; they were coping with the moment-to-moment challenges and unpredictability of new mothering and breastfeeding in a strange place; and they were planning ways of coping in the future when first they returned home and second they returned to a 'normal', usually economically productive life.

### Controlling breastfeeding

Women tended to look ahead and worry about how demand feeding would 'fit in' with their lifestyle. Consequently, they desired to control breastfeeding through placing time constraints upon it and developing a routine; for example Gemma commented that she was somewhat ambivalent about breastfeeding while she was pregnant, 'what put me off was the demand feeding. I've got horses and I like to be out with them. The idea of sitting and feeding all day wasn't me' (P5).

Most women tended to see demand feeding as a short-term endeavour, again emphasising their goal of developing a routine:

> I mean this demand feeding, it's OK to begin with but then I want to get her into some sort of a pattern by one or two months you know, like six to eight weeks or something. Once she's settled into a routine I'll put her cot in the nursery we've got ready.
>
> (Kate, P39)

As may be seen in this quote, a primary goal in relation to mothering the baby centred on progressing the baby towards independence. Development of a routine was a key element of this goal. Another example of a mother who emphasised her desire to impose an early routine may be seen in the following 'staccato' conversation with Pauline. She appeared to see breastfeeding as purely functional for transfer of milk, and not as sensuous, relational or nurturing in any way. She saw expressing and giving formula, and getting the baby used to bottles as early as possible, as the ideal. She rejected the notion of intensive mothering. For her, breastfeeding appeared to be a largely pleasureless, mechanical act centring on the transmission of milk to the baby. Establishment of a routine was a priority:

> I breastfeed because it's better for the baby, it's cheaper, it's convenient ... I mean breastfeeding is all right. It's not something I really enjoy. It's not something I dislike ... it's fine ... I fed my other two for about twelve weeks ... then I'm back to work ... I'll probably do the same this time ... then I switch to formula. I give it to them from quite early on, just to get used to it ... after a few weeks, but I express and get them used to a bottle straight away, because I want them to get used to a bottle and I never had any problem with that ... I like to be quite routined. I do it on demand but try and get them into a routine,

so looking at four hourly really in an ideal world. I think they do suck for comfort and I don't want him sucking for comfort just on me. I'd rather he had a dummy. I've given him a dummy. If he isn't settling I just give him a dummy and see if he just wants comfort or not.

(Pauline, P56)

Pauline saw the need to express milk and give it by bottle and use of formula milk as a part of the routinisation of feeding. As stated, women commonly conceptualised breastfeeding as transferring or delivering breast milk to the baby. This enabled/facilitated an easy step to the provision of breast milk without the baby being at the breast; this may be referred to as breast milk feeding. Expressing breast milk enabled this shift for some. As Van Esterik (1996) states, 'Breast pumps contribute to the medicalization of breastfeeding and emphasize breast milk as a product rather than breastfeeding as a process' (273). Blum (1999) refers to expressing milk to give to the baby as a disembodied approach, with breastfeeding as a relationship vanishing, and mother love being replaced by the pump and breast milk. Jane (P12) illustrated this form of control over breastfeeding as enabling a return to a 'normal life':

Because breast milk is what's advised for the baby's health, I said I'd give it a go. I'll be going back to work full time, so I'd like to be able to express, so if that's all right, but I don't know how easy that's going to be. I'm just concentrating on getting over the first stages first. I'd like to be able ... if I can express I'd like to think I can carry on doing it, depending on how I can work it round. Being able to express obviously makes it more convenient socially and you know having more of a normal life.

(Jane, P12)

This emphasis upon returning to 'normal' by expressing resonates with the findings of Morse and Bottorff (1988) in which they refer to women's knowledge that their infant was receiving breast milk, even in their absence, as the 'door to freedom' (165). The desire to return to 'normal' in relation to one's body and life, as Schmied (1998) argues, parallels dominant discourses around 'control, management and efficiency' (277). Expressing also related to the desire to reduce the intensity of the one-to-one mother-to-baby relationship. This was illustrated by Liz who saw the reduction of intensive mothering as part of a shared parenting endeavour. Shared parenting is increasingly identified by women as a legitimate reason for not exclusively breastfeeding or for bottle feeding (Schmied 1998; Earle 2000; Dykes et al. 2003), 'I'd like to use a breast pump so my partner can take his turn as well. I think that's important. Otherwise you become very isolated together, it's a mother–child thing – breastfeeding' (Liz, P11).

There was a striking sense that transferring the baby to bottles symbolised progress. Indeed, the baby bottle has become such a strong symbol of babyhood in our culture (Henderson et al. 2000) that it is seen as an almost inevitable step in the creation of an independent individual. Some of the women in this study appeared to be uncomfortable with the idea of expressing milk to give by bottle, preferring to give a bottle of formula. This reflects the socio-economic classification of some of the participants, as expressing milk is more prevalent in 'higher occupations' while giving formula milk becomes increasingly prevalent in 'lower occupations' (Hamlyn *et al.* 2002: 18).

Almost without exception, women saw breastfeeding as a relatively short-term project, with three to six months being the longest stated duration. Returning to work was usually given as the reason for discontinuing, 'I'm going back to work in three months time, so I'll probably start bottle feeding then, it'll be easier because I won't be with her all the time' (Carol, P31). The nature of the work was often seen as incompatible with breastfeeding:

> I've got to go back to work in eighteen weeks, so probably I'll breastfeed until then and then change to bottle feeding. I work for an airline so it is not practical to breastfeed. If they gave us longer maternity I would.
>
> (Harriet, P52)

Mandy planned to combine breastfeeding and giving formula milk and then at three months to probably 'progress' to predominantly or all bottle feeding:

> I aim to give him three months start. I've read in the evening you can give a bottle to help them sleep; it's thicker. I've spoken to others with practical experience – they have combined both. Then it may be a bit more difficult after three months, there'll be a few more restrictions, because I'm going back to work.
>
> (Mandy, P25)

Women commonly felt that they needed back-ups to breastfeeding, reflecting their uncertainty and lack of confidence in the notion of exclusive breastfeeding and their desire to shift some of the accountability. The most commonly used backup was a formula supplement:

> I've got some formula at home in case we need it ... but I think both my husband and myself, we feel that if we've actually got something in the house, if we're actually at the stage where the baby's not feeding then we've actually got something to rely on.
>
> (Chloe, P50)

For some women the combination of demand feeding and nipple pain led to feelings of conflict and a desire to protect one's body and turn to bottle feeding; for example Sam was considering bottle feeding as a way of preserving her bodily integrity and reducing the pain:

Well, I've been feeding most of the night and my nipples are very sore, but I'm trying my best to persevere, but I don't know if I'm going to be able to do it. If my nipples crack, I think they might crack, I think I'll go on to the bottle – I'll have to wait and see. I just didn't realise it would be this painful.

(Sam, P19)

Clearly women were heavily influenced by their need to be in control, with linear time placing powerful limits upon their experiences and expectations with regard to breastfeeding. While in hospital they were coping with the past (the birth), the present with all its challenges and transitions, and the future. The future was marked by the temporal notion of time moving on towards the re-establishment of 'normality' with a major part of that being related to returning to paid 'production'. Women's ways of negotiating breastfeeding in hospital therefore related to varying degrees of desire to be in control of their life both in their immediate situations and in the projected longer term.

The preoccupation with return to 'normal activity', control and predictability, combined with women's lack of confidence, contributed to a desire to shift accountability so that women were not solely responsible for nourishing their baby. This desire to avoid being totally accountable for the baby's well-being through breastfeeding, by utilising partial or total bottle feeding, is referred to in other anthropological studies (Maher 1992b; Zeitlyn and Rowsham 1997).

It would be tempting to relate the degree of control women wished to place on to breastfeeding to their like or dislike of it. However, women sometimes reported a positive experience of breastfeeding, but fully intended to introduce bottles. A range of other socio-cultural constraints and influences were inevitably involved. The various forms of supplementing or attenuating breastfeeding enabled women to cope with the present and plan for the future. The bottle, and in particular the bottle of formula milk, was a symbolic marker in that return.

## Moving on

In summary, women's productive projects were largely viewed by the women themselves as transient and temporary, as they planned, even at this early stage, for resumption of their 'normal' productive lives with return to paid employment being a central consideration. There were four dimensions to women's productive projects: those of providing, supplying, demanding and controlling. However, most women expressed a mistrust in the efficacy of their bodies, conceptualising themselves as machines. Women referred to the unpredictable way in which their babies 'demanded' breast milk and thereby breached their once-ordered temporal boundaries. In addition, the baby made indentations into their spatial and bodily boundaries. Women often felt wary of their baby 'depending' upon them in this way.

It was particularly striking that women spoke repeatedly about breastfeeding as if it were simply breast milk feeding. There was rarely a notion of relationality with the baby. It seems, then, unsurprising that the task was seen as demanding, as the act of breastfeeding was understood as a one-way transfer of nutrition. Without the two-way reciprocity of a relationship, the act of providing for another is likely to be experienced as depleting. While the hospital culture in itself could not account for women's perceptions of their bodies and bodily functions, it played a reinforcing role. The combination of lack of confidence, fear of chaos, unpredictability and sense of planning for the future led to women trying to maintain their boundaries and control breastfeeding, often through making plans to incorporate 'bottles' of either expressed milk or formula milk. This was commonly seen as a necessary and desirable progression towards independence for mother and child, and a return to normality. In the next chapter I draw parallels between the productive projects of breastfeeding women and those of midwives.

# Chapter 5

# 'Time to care'

## Midwifery work at the end of the medical production line

### Introduction

In this chapter I focus upon the working conditions for hospital midwives, with the metaphor of the factory, with its notions of production, demand and efficient supply, against linear time, being central to their experiences. I highlight midwives as the main group of people with whom women engage while in hospital and illustrate ways in which they negotiate and indeed 'process' their work, given the enormous constraints upon them. The impact of midwives' ways of working in hospital upon the experiences of women is illustrated.

There are four main ways through which people experience situations: temporality, spaciality, corporeality and relationality (Merleau-Ponty 1962). While the main focus in this section is upon relational aspects of women's experiences, time, space and the body were intricately interwoven for both mothers and midwives. Taking this into account, I contextualise the work by describing the cultural settings in which midwives are coping (or not) with 'caring'. To support this contextualisation I draw upon relevant theory with regard to caring/uncaring encounters but also upon research that highlights the constraints upon midwives and nurses within institutionalised health care settings.

I first refer to encounters in which there was a general failure to 'take time' and 'touch base'. I define 'touching base', a metaphor used by one of the participants, as 'touching the personal experience of another'. I describe ways in which time was 'taken' away from midwives and mothers. I then refer to encounters in which midwives took time and touched base with women, in that they made ways of 'finding time' to facilitate positive relationships with women.

### The nature of encounters

With regard to relational aspects of women's experiences, a range of interchangeable and overlapping terms may be utilised to describe encounters with healthcare staff, for example: supportive/unsupportive (Gill 2001; Lugina *et al.* 2001), caring/uncaring (Woodward 2000), empowering/disempowering (Halldorsdottir and Karlsdottir 1996a), helpful/unhelpful (Chen *et al.* 2001), sensitive/insensitive

(Mozingo *et al.* 2000), facilitative/inhibitive (Fenwick *et al.* 2000, 2001). Some authors utilise one term, for example support, to encompass caring along with other desirable aspects within encounters and relationships. For example, Sarafino (1994) highlights five types of essential social support: 'emotional support' (caring and empathy); 'esteem support' (positive regard by others, agreement and encouragement); 'instrumental support' (practical assistance); 'informational support' (provision of information); and 'network support' (company and membership of a group with common interests) (103).

There is also a vast literature on communications in healthcare settings, some of which overlaps considerably with the above, for example Kirkham (1983, 1989, 1993, 1997a). Effective communication may be seen simply as a means of conveying information but is more recently being described in its fundamental links with relationships in healthcare settings (Kirkham 2000a, 2000b; Edwards 2001, 2005). However, an encounter may arguably still be considered caring even if a relationship has not been established. Finally, there is a growing literature on the influence of the culture/environment upon healthcare workers' abilities to support service-users (Kirkham 1999; Woodward 2000; Kirkham and Stapleton 2001b; Ball *et al.* 2002; Hughes *et al.* 2002; Hunter 2002, 2004, 2005; Deery 2003, 2005).

As I reflected on this literature in relation to the data, I realised the possible contradictions inherent in some of these classifications when applied to women starting out as new mothers and embarking upon the experience of breastfeeding. The methodology I used enabled me to elicit from mothers, and to a lesser extent from midwives, how they felt about the nature of their encounters with each other. However, I was also able to observe the encounters, resulting in a synthesis of perspectives: the mothers', the midwives' and my own. I therefore move beyond describing what is *said* to include what is *done*. As an observer, I watched encounters in which the information given regarding breastfeeding was misleading and counterproductive to the effective establishment and maintenance of breastfeeding. However, these encounters, if conducted in a pleasant and encouraging way, might be perceived by women as supportive. In contrast, midwives might provide information that was useful for the establishment of breastfeeding, but because it was delivered in a disconnected, routine and unfriendly manner it may have been discouraging for women. Thus encounters could be encouraging but not enabling to effective breastfeeding, or potentially helpful in relation to breastfeeding but generally discouraging.

Fenwick *et al.*'s (1999, 2000, 2001) research on facilitative and inhibitive nursing actions was very relevant to the data I generated. Their research was conducted in an Australian neonatal unit and involved tape recording interactions between nurses and parents in addition to conducting interviews with both groups. They found that the verbal exchanges between nurse and mother influenced a woman's confidence, sense of control and her feelings of connection with her infant. They identified two types of nursing behaviour, with the first described as 'facilitative nursing action', which women felt helped them to feel connected with their babies (Fenwick *et al.* 2000: 197). This involved the use of positive language which expressed care, support and interest in parents with 'chatting' and using personal experience in a sensitive way being used as a strategy through which positive interactions were initiated, maintained and enhanced (Fenwick *et al.* 2001: 253). Mothers, when interviewed, were more interested in how things were said than what was being said (Fenwick *et al.* 2001: 588). The other two key facilitative nursing actions involved nurses 'walking beside the mother', that is working with the mother, encouraging her and sharing information with her, and 'respecting the woman's status as a mother', that is listening, negotiating, sharing decisions and giving the mother space (Fenwick *et al.* 2000: 199).

The second type of nursing behaviour, described as 'inhibitive nursing action', reflected a more authoritarian style of approach (Fenwick *et al.* 2000: 197). It included nurses maintaining their position as expert, maintaining control, directing care, supervising and directing the mother, dismissing women's skills, showing preoccupation with protecting the infant, and guarding safety. The approach was autocratic, didactic, clinical, robotic, cold and unfriendly and the language was medical and technical (Fenwick *et al.* 2000). Meticulous rituals were performed and there was a felt power differential with women feeling chastised, naughty and child-like. Women described how this nursing behaviour made them feel defensive and helpless, heightened their sense of isolation and separation from their infant and constrained them in their mothering role and relationship with the baby (Fenwick *et al.* 2000, 2001). This contribution to caring theory recognises that the development of a trusting relationship is highly desirable, but it illustrates that a single encounter in itself can be positive or highly negative to the way a woman feels. This provides an important perspective because in reality in many practice-based situations, encounters are short-lived and not based on an intimate, therapeutic or intense relationship that has developed over a considerable period of time.

The fertility clinic ethnography described by Allan (2001) further illuminates issues in relation to the short-term encounter. She argues that caring in this context is not based on an intense relationship but on practical, skilled support accompanied by 'emotional awareness' (51). The women wanted nurses to *know* what they were going through and to *be there* when they were needed. In contrast, women described 'emotional distance' as the nurse acting practically for the patients but not responding at times when they expressed emotional distress. These nurses were seen to be 'caring for the clinic' rather than the patients (54). Allan (2001) argues that good enough nursing allows nurses enough distance to be able to cope with the emotional difficulties inherent in their work and that, provided they are able to respond to emotional needs when expressed, patients accept this care as 'good enough' (57). This perspective has enabled me to avoid placing my own ideals upon the data in terms of relational aspects of encounters and rather to accept that by the time women have come through the fragmented care systems within western maternity services, they are unlikely to voice any sense of loss at not having a deep relationship with midwives. They may be satisfied with 'good enough' care during this final phase in their journey through the maternity service. This does not justify the way things are but it assists in understanding data based on brief encounters. Nevertheless, many of the experiences of the women in my study illustrated that the care they received was not 'good enough' for them and it is upon this that I first focus.

## The culture of caring

Much of the research on caring has little to say on the context of care and its impact upon midwives' ways of working. However, the culture through which women learn to breastfeed and midwives work is crucial. It plays a key role in how women cope with their emotions, their change of role and learning to breast-feed, and how midwives cope with their emotions and role. The importance of a political and cultural awareness of the context within which midwives work is highlighted by Davis-Floyd (1992) and Davis-Floyd and St John (1998) in the US, and Kirkham (1999), Kirkham and Stapleton (2001b) and Ball *et al.* (2002) in the UK. These authors powerfully illustrate aspects of the maternity hospital setting with its techno-medical culture and hierarchical, separatist, gendered and indeed oppressive systems.

There is also a growing literature on nurses' and midwives' coping behaviours within institutions and the negative effects of these behaviours on service users and indeed themselves. The seminal work of Menzies (1960, 1970) relates to the ways in which nursing organisation and practice influences the development of behaviours. Her study within the UK hospital nursing system reflects the anxieties and tensions inherent in hospital-based work. Drawing on psychoanalytical theory, she refers to the development of nursing 'social defence' techniques (11). These include task-orientation, thus limiting relationship-building with 'patients' and indeed colleagues; depersonalisation of the individual patient; detachment and denial of the nurse's feelings; and avoidance of change. She argues that these defences limit the capacity to engage in creative, symbolic and abstract thought and conceptualisation and sense of one's own potential. Thus the institution of the hospital and its activities create a way of being and working for health staff that exacerbates the negative effects upon them and in turn the service users.

The widely quoted work of Hochschild (1979) on emotional labour and emotion management extends that of Menzies in that she refers to the ways in which social ordering and expectations actually affect what people allow themselves to feel, that is 'feeling rules' (551), and how social factors affect what people actually think and do about what they feel. The latter results in 'emotion management' (551). While she refers to this management of feelings in relation to air hostesses, it is highly applicable to midwives. This connection with midwives is made by Hunter (2001, 2002, 2004, 2005) who extensively explored how midwives experience and manage emotion in their work. Hunter (2002) was able to study midwives' 'emotion work' in the hospital setting and compare this with those emotions generated and managed within the community setting.

Hunter (2002, 2004, 2005) refers to emotion work as the work involved in managing feelings in the self and others. The opportunity for Hunter to study the differences between hospital and community was provided by a recent integration of the maternity service, with midwives now entering both settings but remembering their original place of work. Hunter does not refer to Foucault, but she perhaps could have done in that the self-disciplining and regulation of bodies seems to link closely with the concept of emotion work. As Frank (1990) argues, 'panopticism takes on a new intensity in emotional labour' (159).

A similar opportunity to compare both community and hospital settings was described by Lock in her phenomenological study with Australian women taking early postnatal discharge (Lock 1999; Lock and Gibb 2003). While her focus was primarily upon the experience of women, she too was able to fortuitously focus upon the difference between midwifery practice at home and in hospital by the same midwives. While neither author refers to each other, some of their conclusions are striking in their similarity, as I will now highlight.

Hunter (2002, 2004, 2005) argues that there are several contributory factors to the emotion work of hospital midwives. The most profound source stems from a lack of congruence between beliefs and ideals and the reality of practice within a discipline that has many contradictory values. This was particularly the case for students and recently qualified midwives. This creates dissonance. Hunter (2002, 2004, 2005) argues that an increase in dissonance relates, in part, to the widely acclaimed 'new midwifery' philosophy (Page 2000) with its 'ideal' low-tech, women-centred, one-to-one focus. This contrasts with the 'reality' of a highly medicalised, fragmented and frequently interrupted form of institutional midwifery still evident in many UK maternity units. The hospital midwife is also bound by the implicit and explicit rules of the organisation and her occupational autonomy is thereby seriously limited. This results in the midwife being clearly 'with institution' rather than 'with woman' (Hunter 2004: 261), as also noted by others (Lock 1999; Allan 2001; Kirkham and Stapleton 2001b; Shallow 2001a, 2001b, 2001c, 2001d, Ball *et al.* 2002; Deery 2003, 2005; Lock and Gibb 2003).

Hunter (2002, 2004, 2005) highlights the ways in which hospital midwives engage in emotion work. One of the strategies involves task orientation and routinisation in an attempt to impose control and keep workloads manageable. The midwife becomes emotionally gratified by getting through the work, completing tasks and handing over to the next shift, thus providing her with a sense that the story has ended. In contrast, community work is more emotionally gratifying through relationships, and the story continues rather than ending. To cope with the emotion work, midwives engage in impression management, involving controlling and hiding of emotions. They develop self-protective barriers and boundaries in which they are able to enter a disengaged state of withdrawal and distancing when overwhelmed emotionally.

While Hunter (2002, 2004, 2005) is careful to avoid blurring emotion work with caring, the effects of emotion work upon encounters between midwives and mothers become apparent. Both Lock and Gibb (2003) and Hunter (2002, 2004,

2005) highlight fundamental differences between the hospital and home encounter. In the home there was an opportunity for relationality and the midwife had more occupational autonomy (Lock and Gibb 2003; Hunter 2002, 2004, 2005). Talk at home was more likely to be woman-initiated, as this was her territory, not the midwife's (Lock and Gibb 2004). The encounters at home took on a more informal, social and reciprocal nature with more chatter and use of self by midwives (Lock and Gibb 2003; Hunter 2002, 2004, 2005).

Lock and Gibb (2003) refer to the midwife having temporal autonomy in the home, with the mothers being highly aware that they had the midwife one-to-one for a period of uninterrupted time. Thus time at home was prescribed by the needs of the woman, not the institution. It becomes clear, then, that while institutions and their rules do encroach upon community midwifery, particularly in integrated services (Edwards 2001, 2005; Hunter 2002, 2004, 2005), the 'power of place' (Lock and Gibb 2003) upon midwives' emotion work and resulting approach to women is tangible and significant (132).

Lipsky's (1980) work is particularly illuminating with regard to the ways in which public service workers process work. He explored the working practices of public service workers within 'street level bureaucracies', i.e. schools, police, welfare departments and other agencies that provide a dispensatory service to the public (xi). Staff within these organisations are placed in a situation whereby the requirements of their jobs make it impossible for them to achieve their ideal conceptions of the job. Due to the volume of work, restricted resources and unpredictability, they develop 'modes of mass production' that enable them to process clients through the system most effectively (xii). This inevitably involves the development of strategies to ration and routinise work, alter their expectations of the job and in some cases stereotype and/or select some clients for which they provide the ideal service, thus providing themselves with a limited form of job satisfaction.

Kaplan *et al.* (1996) illustrated similar effects upon encounters with clients in healthcare situations where health professionals are coping with high volumes of work. They established a clear link between volume of work, levels of occupational autonomy and, in turn, participatory styles in medical doctors. They concluded, 'if a sense of personal autonomy is related to a more participatory style, then those physicians who view themselves as more able to control their practice environment may show a more flexible style with their patients' (503).

Low levels of occupational autonomy are strongly related to occupational stress with inevitable consequences for service users. Indeed, occupational stress is maximised in situations where high pressure is combined with low levels of control/autonomy over working conditions (Brunner 1996; Syme 1996; Tarlov 1996). The relationship between low occupational autonomy and high levels of stress and burnout has been identified in midwifery contexts (Sandall 1997; Mackin and Sinclair 1999; Shallow 2001c; Ball *et al.* 2002), as has the relationship between inability to experience relationality with women and stress and burnout (Sandall 1997; Shallow 2001b; Ball *et al.* 2002). In contrast, high levels of occupational autonomy and opportunity for relationality with women increase satisfaction and morale in midwifery work (Sandall 1997, Hunter 1999, 2002; Stevens and McCourt 2002b).

The complex and detrimental combination of low occupational autonomy, ideological dissonance and absence of relationality in midwifery work cannot be separated from the power of linear time upon midwives, as I illustrate with the data I present. The critical ethnography of nursing by Street (1992) is particularly useful in relation to my growing awareness of the tyranny of linear time upon midwives. She refers to the work of Foucault (1977) in stating that 'timetables, whether rigidly imposed or tacitly agreed upon, penetrate the rhythms of the body, disciplining and controlling them' (109). She refers to the ways in which times, rhythms and manoeuvres turn hospital nurses' bodies into efficient machines. She describes the discipline and subjugation of nurses' bodies through a multiplicity of processes within hospitals. These range from unsociable shifts, rigid timetables, requirement to eat and drink at specific times in specific places, and wearing of restrictive uniforms. She describes the regulated and disciplined way in which they are trained to conduct tasks such as making beds with required efficiency, economy and synchronisation of movement. Under these circumstances activities centre around saving time and using time efficiently. In addition, Street (1992) refers to the stress placed on nurses when trying to make clinical judgements under the pressure of constantly changing and unpredictable scenarios.

The collective nursing ethnographies of Varcoe et al. (2003) also illustrate the continuing nature of the culture of 'efficient processing' (962), with nurses maintaining a culture in which colleagues are valued for their emotional strength and efficiency. Nurses passively accept and embrace an 'ideology of scarcity' (964) related to inadequacies of time, money and staffing. The notion of efficient use of time is also highlighted in midwifery contexts (Kirkham and Stapleton 2001a; Ball et al. 2002; Stapleton et al. 2002b).

## Failing to take time and 'touch base'

In this section, I describe negative aspects of the midwife–mother interactions. Women commonly started their short postnatal journey following a medicalised birth. They were then subjected to a range of rituals and procedures, mechanistic language and a reductionist approach to breastfeeding support. Reference to breastfeeding was often disconnected from the woman's birth experience, previous experience, life in general, her agenda and metaphorically from her body. Women tended to describe their encounters with midwives as representing a 'failure to touch base'. This was compounded by lack of information, misinformation, conflicting advice and unhelpful use of personal experience. The encounters generally failed to meet women's needs for confidence-building, encouragement, emotional, practical and informational support.

In Chapter 3, I described the settings in which midwives were working and mothers breastfeeding. The ways of working resembled production-line conditions and, like the work of factory staff, midwifery work was spatially restricted, segmented, repetitive and constrained by clock time (Menzies 1960; Forman 1989; Street 1992). There were powerful constraints of linear time upon midwives' bodies, as they were tied into a system in which their daily work centred upon urgency and meeting unrealistic deadlines. Almost every midwife I spoke to referred to the pressure of racing against time. Midwives faced constant unpredictability in that at any moment either they or a colleague could be called to cover delivery suite. This would require rapid reorientation of the 'sent' individual and reorganisation by remaining staff who would suddenly be left one or two members of staff short. Emergencies could arise at any time, particularly with the antenatal women, creating more unpredictability. This unpredictability meant that, whether busy or not, there was pressure to get through the work in case circumstances changed. This contributed to a rushed and fragmented approach to care as referred to by others (Ball 1994; Kirkham 1999; Kirkham and Stapleton 2000; Ball *et al.* 2002).

The mode of communication I most commonly observed with regard to breastfeeding was one of issuing advice in a monologic manner according to a pre-set agenda. There appeared to be little attempt to listen to the woman, to come to know her expectations, to ascertain what she already knew or to learn about how breastfeeding fitted in with her life and recent birthing. This conforms with other critiques of postnatal care (Ball 1994; Lomax and Robinson 1996; Bondas-Salonen 1998; Garcia *et al.* 1998; Lavender *et al.* 2000; Singh and Newburn 2000). Midwives commonly approached women with an authoritative air and a knowledge that seemed to be owned by them. They thus displayed the characteristic mode of communication within the techno-medical model in which the professional is assumed to have the expert and authoritative knowledge and the mother to be a passive recipient or receptacle of the wisdom instilled (Jordan 1997; Edwards 2000, 2005). This relates to Freire's (1972) notion of depositing knowledge while the recipient is simply a depository.

This way of communicating left women in a state of tension between dependence on health professionals for information and advice and their need to be in touch with signals from both their bodies and their babies. This inevitably undermined their confidence. The inequality in power created by the midwives' approaches rendered effective dialogue, a two-way process between equals, almost impossible to fulfil, as also reported by Kirkham (1993) and Stapleton *et al.* (2002b).

In Chapter 4, I highlighted ways in which women experienced a lack of confidence and control with regard to breastfeeding that related in part to current and projected concerns about their productivity and the unpredictability and time-consuming nature of breastfeeding. They sought to regain control over the erosion of their temporal and spatial boundaries in a range of ways. Like that of the women, the midwives' work centred upon productivity and output. They utilised physical and emotional strategies to get through the work in ways that enabled them to partially control for the general unpredictability and temporal pressures.

To illustrate the nature of encounters within this setting, I discuss the organising themes of 'communicating temporal pressure', 'rituals, routines and procedures', 'disconnected encounters', 'managing breastfeeding' and 'rationing information'.

### Communicating pressure

Midwives' ways of working and communicating reflected the ongoing pressures created by linear time constraints and unpredictability. Midwives communicated a powerful sense of urgency that led to rushed and disconnected communications. The women referred to the pressures on midwives: 'They seem to be pressured, panicking and anxious' (Bryony, P7): 'The midwives seem to be, you know ... um ... spread very thinly and they don't have much time' (Alison, P38). Women disliked receiving inadequate staff time and availability and feeling rushed, as referred to in related studies (Tarkka and Paunonen 1996; Bondas-Salonen 1998; Bowes and Domokos 1998; Svedulf *et al.* 1998; Tarkka *et al.* 1998; Vogel and Mitchell 1998; Whelan and Lupton 1998; Lock 1999; Hoddinott and Pill 2000; Hauck *et al.* 2002; Hong *et al.* 2003). Women felt that their needs were only petty and insignificant in the grand scheme of things and that to call a busy midwife for breastfeeding was to 'drag her away' from an important or urgent task:

> I mean, you don't like bothering people because I know that they are SO SO busy. You know, they keep saying buzz us to lift him out of the crib for you, because he's so heavy as well. But I mean ... you know ... um ... it's dragging them away from somebody who has just given birth, or ... whatever. I just won't ... I mean something like lifting him out of the crib seems so ... petty really, to be asking them that.
>
> (Sue, P29 – first-day post-Caesarean section)

As a result of their awareness of the midwives' pressure and busyness, women tended to struggle on, quietly recognising that asking for support or information was to request midwifery time. Under these busy conditions, mothers were reluctant to ask for help, findings that resonate with those of Kirkham and Stapleton (2001b), and Bowes and Domokos (1998). Only some women were able to secure midwives' time, leaving women who were less confident and assertive particularly silent. The more silent women tended to be those from lower income groups and therefore I saw the inverse care law (Lipsky 1980; Townsend and Davidson 1992) in operation. This has also been highlighted within maternity care settings by Kirkham *et al.* (2002b). On both sites, midwives commonly told women that they would come back later but I rarely saw this happen:

*Francesca (MW28):*   How's the breastfeeding going?
*Annie (P42):*   My nipples are sore.
*Francesca:*   Can I have a look? *(Annie showed her nipples.)* Right, well you may feel some tenderness, but we don't want them to

|        |                                                        |
|--------|--------------------------------------------------------|
|        | get cracked and bleeding. When you next feed can you give |
|        | us a shout and I'll check the position for you.        |
| *Annie:* | Yeah, OK.                                            |

Women made excuses for the midwives and generally recognised the constraints upon them, as illustrated by Louise (P14). Although Louise was highly dissatisfied with the nature of her encounters with midwives, she did not blame them as individuals: rather she highlighted problems with the system and its effect upon midwives making them busy, pressured and stressed, 'I mean it's not their fault, the midwives, they want to give but they just can't. It's not their fault; it's the pressure here; with the best will in the world they can't do it' (Louise, P14). This sympathy expressed by several of the women towards midwives was also reported by Kirkham and Stapleton (2001b). Indeed Kirkham and Stapleton (2001b) state, 'a number of service users recognised midwives as an oppressed group' (147).

In order to test to see whether midwives' approaches changed when the wards were quiet I followed the same midwives through during busy and quiet periods. I became aware that while a few midwives adjusted their pace depending on the busyness, most adopted the busy mode whatever the ward state. This maintenance of 'busy mode' in hospital regardless of number of women to care for resonates with the findings of Lock and Gibb (2003). The lack of slowing of pace in quieter periods probably relates in part to the sense that at any moment a member of staff could be moved, immediately changing the distribution of workload. Additionally, once midwives have developed a particular way of engaging with women, it becomes a patterned form of behaviour that is difficult to change.

I referred to the unpredictable working conditions for the midwives from their perspective in Chapter 3, but this was also reported by the women:

> They're all so busy. There don't seem to be a lot of staff, they're rushed off their feet, they really are. There was one day this week when it wasn't so busy ... um ... a few had been discharged and they had more time to spend with you, but like the other night, there were that many people coming in and out, people delivering, they don't have time to do anything. It seems like a few staff are trying to see to a lot of people. I suppose they never know how busy they're going to be. I mean, on a ward where they have booked operations it's different, but here you don't know who's going to have a baby.
>
> (Vicky, P30)

Here Vicky alluded to the notion of mass processing of women described by Lipsky (1980) in relation to public sector workers. The erratic and serendipitous nature of care led to some women being completely overlooked; for example Annette (P58) was being looked after by one midwife who was later sent elsewhere so no one saw her for most of the first day. Annette appeared to have a low sense of confidence in breastfeeding. By day two she had decided to bottle feed and declined being interviewed. I discussed this with Anthea (MW25):

F:                        Do you know why Annette stopped breastfeeding?
Anthea (MW25):   No, we just came on in the morning and she'd changed to bottle feeding. She got a bit missed yesterday, because Sandy [MW30] had to go to theatre and no one really got to see the ladies in her bay until after handover, so her baby hadn't really fed properly since 10pm the night before. Anyway, we took her temperature and she was a bit cold and we did a BM which was 2.5, which wasn't bad, so we warmed her up and then she fed better, when she was warmer. But in the night she gave up breastfeeding.

Clearly, the combination of temporal pressure and unpredictability set the scene for a series of encounters with women that were largely inadequate in meeting their needs. The most striking manifestation of emotion management occurred through the use of rituals, routines and procedures, to which I now turn.

### Rituals, routines and procedures

A substantial part of the activity conducted on the postnatal ward centred around ritualistic performance of procedures. There is lack of consensus as to what a ritual actually involves (Philpin 2002), but I adopt an anthropological definition. Anthropologist Davis-Floyd (1992) defines a ritual as a 'patterned, repetitive, and symbolic enactment of a cultural belief or value' (8):

> In all cultures, people use repetitive rituals to provide themselves with a sense of order, stability, and control. In professions like medicine, where chaos and uncertainty pervade daily practice, cleaving to ritualistic routines in which they can demonstrate clear competence can hold fear at bay and give practitioners a much-valued sense of confidence and control over what are often very uncertain outcomes.
>
> (Davis-Floyd and St John 1998: 32)

Menzies (1960) refers to ritual task-performance as a mechanism for reducing the anxiety created by the emotive and unpredictable nature of hospital nursing, although she notes that these defence mechanisms often increase rather than reduce anxiety in the long term. Health workers' adherence to ritual activity was illustrated by Davies and Atkinson (1991) in an ethnographic study of a cohort of nurses during early clinical placements on their midwifery course. The authors described 'doing the obs' as a coping strategy for dealing with feelings of strangeness, inadequacy and low self-esteem. This ritual, they argue, has become the exclusive responsibility of the nurse. Both Menzies (1960) and Davies and Atkinson (1991) note that this routinised behaviour forms a very early part of the socialisation of student nurses within the hospital environment.

Fox (1989) likewise refers to the turning of obstetrics into a mechanical act and a time-bound process that assists the 'caregiver' to cope with her/his inner turmoil with time being reduced from a 'subjective experience to a rational, intelligible, measurable means of orientation' (126). She argues that obstetric 'caregivers' protect themselves by introducing an orderliness to the process, invoking feelings of being in control over the painful issues of life and death and their own helplessness:

> This painful state is literally covered over by the ceaseless demands and absorbing routines of medical practice. There is not time to linger over what's past: onward to new problems, new patients, new treatments. The present is thus materialized, fuelled with concrete evidence of one's productivity.
>
> (126)

This emphasis upon the place of routinised and ritual behaviour in coping with anxiety and giving people a feeling of being in control, especially in the face of ambiguity, unpredictability and aversive situations, is being increasingly recognised in public service (Lipsky 1980) and health settings (Kirkham 1989; Davies and Atkinson 1991; Ball 1994; Hunt and Symonds 1995; Begley 2001; Hunter 2002, 2004, 2005; Philpin 2002; Waterworth 2003). In terms of the effects on recipients of care, as Hunt and Symonds (1995) state, 'women's wants, needs and even rights are swallowed up in procedures and routines' (129). The passivity created by the system is highlighted by Kirkham (1989) who describes the 'medicalized nature of the setting' in which 'patients' are 'processed', with rules and routines emphasising their role as 'passive work objects' (131).

The women I interviewed and observed had had many aspects of their pregnant and labouring bodies subjected to measurement such as weighing the mother, ultrasound measurement of the fetus and counting fetal movements. This measurement then reached a climax in the labouring mother, when every aspect of her progress was charted meticulously on a partogram and judged against linear time; for example the dilatation of her cervix in centimetres, the frequency and length of her contractions. Finally women arrived on to the postnatal ward, only to be introduced to a new set of routines, with the potential to perpetuate their perception of themselves as passive recipients of 'care' and prone to deficiencies, as expressed in their beliefs about their milk. To illustrate the organising theme of rituals, routines and procedures I refer to three aspects of this theme: the 'postnatal check'; 'ritual removal of medical attachments'; and 'ticking tasks off'.

The postnatal examination or check constituted the dominant procedure on the wards. It is not my purpose to suggest the appropriateness or otherwise of this procedure or to analyse in depth the content of the postnatal examinations. However, as the 'check' often set the 'scene' for subsequent communications, to include providing women with breastfeeding support, it requires a mention. The postnatal check was usually conducted in an asymmetrical manner, also referred to by Lomax and Robinson (1996), with the midwife very much controlling the agenda. In most cases there was a brief discussion commenced by an open question, such as 'what kind of night did you have?' Conversation which preceded the postnatal check was closed down with an indication that the 'business' was about to commence, with comments such as 'right I'll just check you over now', or 'I'll just wash my hands then I'll sort you out', a finding also reported by Lomax and Robinson (1996). In some cases, when the ward was busy, the midwife launched straight into the check:

*Tina (MW1):*  I'll just check your temperature and pulse *(proceeded to do so).*
                  Breasts nice and soft?
*Bev (P2):*     Yes fine
*Tina:*         Not sore anywhere?
*Bev:*          No
*Tina:*         Getting him on properly?
*Bev:*          Yes
*Tina:*         Legs all right?
*Bev:*          Fine
*Tina:*         Can I just feel your tummy?
                  *(Mother wriggled down the bed and lifted up her nighty).*
*Tina:*         OK, that's nice and firm. How's your loss?
*Bev:*          It's like a period ... um ... sort of red.
*Tina:*         Have you passed any clots?
*Bev:*          No
*Tina:*         Appetite OK?
*Bev:*          Yes
*Tina:*         Bowels and waterworks?
*Bev:*          All right
*Tina:*         Sleeping OK?
*Bev:*          Yes, I slept well last night
*Tina:*         Anything you want to ask?
*Bev:*          When will I be able to go home?
*Tina:*         Probably tomorrow if all's well

This encounter was conducted in a highly directive, monologic, midwife-led way, full of closed and leading questions with little scope for discussion. This type of communication, which clearly centred upon a predetermined agenda, resonates with the findings of others (Bondas-Salonen 1998; Kirkham and Stapleton 2001a; Stapleton *et al.* 2002d). The postnatal checks were often concluded by the midwife taking up a standing position behind the mother's table and carefully concentrating on the records. This giving of a clear message, 'I'm concentrating, do not disturb', was referred to in Kirkham's (1993) labour ward study (1) and subsequent research (Kirkham and Stapleton 2001a; Stapleton *et al.* 2002b).

The predominance of the postnatal check on both sites emphasised what appeared to be the central role of the midwife in monitoring and checking the woman and baby for problems which should then be corrected, as highlighted in related studies (Ball 1994; Edwards 2000, 2005; Kirkham and Stapleton 2001a). Indeed, Stapleton *et al.* (2002d) refer to the midwife as seeing the woman as a 'body to be thoroughly and appropriately checked' (395). Most women appeared to be resigned to the checking role of the midwife and therefore I saw little questioning or resistance. This emphasis upon checking has come to be seen as a central role of midwives by women in their care, as highlighted by others (Fleming 1998a; Leach *et al.* 1998).

At a time when women were undergoing a major life transition to that of mother of a first or new baby, women who had had a Caesarean section were subjected to a ritual removal of the various tubes inserted during the Caesarean section. The removal of the tubes which symbolically connect the women to the medical system appeared to give the midwives a sense of achievement and progress, a sense of a job well done. Interactions around breastfeeding were often interspersed with post-operative routines:

| | |
|---|---|
| *Di (MW18):* | *(arrived and looked at the baby in the cot)* Has he gone back to sleep? |
| *Veronica (P27):* | Yes |
| *Di:* | Right my love, we'll give you a suppository, for the pain, then we'll get you in the bath, then we'll put him on the breast – how does that sound? |
| *Veronica:* | Um ... fine, thanks |
| *Di:* | Right my love. How are you feeling? |
| *Veronica:* | Um, my nipples are sore |
| *Di:* | Oh, we'll need to check he's on properly when he goes on, OK? |
| *Veronica:* | Yes, thanks |
| *Di:* | Right, can you just turn onto your left side and I'll give you this suppository. *(Mother turned onto her side.)* |
| *Di:* | That's it, all right you'll just feel me inserting it now. *(Proceeded to give her a suppository.)* All right? |
| *Veronica:* | Yes |
| *Di:* | *(Went to wash her hands and returned)* We'll take the drip down, take your catheter out, sit you up and you'll feel a new woman *(laughs).* *(Veronica laughed. The baby cried.)* |
| *Di:* | We're coming! Lets look at your nipples. *(Mother opened her nighty.)* Mmm, they don't look sore. OK, OK, come on *(to the baby). (Lifted the baby to the mother who was on her side. Holding the baby and the mother's breast she 'connected' the two):* Right, so point the nipple to nose, then you'll see more of areola above than below, the top lip is curled back see and the bottom lip turned down. Look you can see his lips? |

| | |
|---|---|
| *Veronica:* | It doesn't feel sore now he's on, it's when he goes on. |
| *Di:* | OK, um, I'll pop back in a minute |
| *Di:* | *(a few minutes later)* How's he doing? I'll give you a pack of leaflets – we'll go through those when we discharge you. *(Veronica put the leaflets away and the midwife went again. No further reference was made to the leaflets.)* *(A few minutes later.)* |
| *Di:* | How does it feel now? Any soreness? *(Referring to the breast-feeding.)* |
| *Veronica:* | Oh it's all right now. It's just when he goes on. He's just sucking and sucking. |
| *Di:* | See how he's slipped off a little – he's just sucking on the end of your nipple, that's when you'll get a bit sore. *(Baby came off and cried.)* I'll just take a sample from the catheter and then take it out. *(Proceeded to take her catheter out and went off with it.)* *(A few minutes later.)* |
| *Di:* | Right, I think we'll try the other side. You are a hungry boy – you are a hungry lad aren't you. Right, point your nipple upwards. *(She helped the baby onto the other side and sat with the mother for a few minutes and then the baby came off.)* |
| *Di:* | Well, we can't say he hasn't had a good feed. Right, if you could just turn onto your back a bit, I'll take your drip down and your dressing off. *(Then with accompanying explanation, she removed the intravenous infusion and then the dressing, etc. and asked the care assistant to take her for a shower.)* When you come back from the shower, we'll pop him next to you again. *(A few minutes later the care assistant came and took Veronica for a shower.)* |

Again, once routine procedures had been completed the midwives would stand by the bed and complete their forms, tick boxes, etc. Midwives throughout their work illustrated their central and instrumental preoccupation with getting tasks completed and ticking boxes. This related to the pressures upon their time and to the unpredictability. It was also a powerful manifestation of task-related behaviour. This was also referred to by women, as was vividly illustrated in my interview with Louise:

> They were very busy yesterday. I'd sort of approached her (the midwife) with a sample and then all of a sudden – ooh I'll do all your notes while you're here sort of thing *(laughs)*. She was taking her opportunity. I mean nobody spoke to me then all afternoon, which was fine – I didn't need anything and I would have called if I had needed anything. I think it was the pressure that had contributed, that she thought I'll get all this done, you know I don't know

if there was a box that she had to tick, to say that she had covered everything. To me she seemed to be only interested in checking my pulse, filling all her forms out and ticking the boxes. I mean I think that whoever is looking after you should come at least twice a day and say 'how are you doing' and 'how are you getting on'; you know just check that everything is going all right. I got the impression that it was more 'oh I'll get this done'. I mean they should at least touch base with you once or twice a day. The night staff didn't speak to me, they were so busy and now two days have gone by.

(Louise, P14)

Louise clearly emphasised the importance of midwives 'touching base' with women. While I was interviewing her, a midwife, Shannon, arrived and announced, 'I'm going to take this down for you [patient-controlled analgesia – PCA] and I'm going to give you a suppository if you don't mind – that's good pain relief for you, all right?' (Shannon MW6). During the two days I observed Louise she highlighted the issues for me in a profound way, not simply with language but with eye contact and body language. She was showing me as well as telling me. I wrote in my field notes:

I feel a strange sense of connection with Louise. She's watching me as I watch her. We're both aware of the same things. We're watching together as people come and go, rarely touching base, rarely listening, working their way through the tasks and ticking things off. We make frequent eye contact as each person approaches her one-by-one with clip board, notebook or case notes in hand – dedicated to task. There's a sense that we understand each other's situation. She's silently highlighting the issues for me as they occur and then as we meet and talk she's summarising for me, constructing the story for me. I feel that closeness to her that I know the midwives here can't have. I want to reach out to her and meet her needs, but I know she'll be all right. I know she has an inner knowing and strength through deep reflection on her first birth, mothering and feeding experience. I know she empathises with me too. I know she wants me to see what it is like for women here and to lay bare the deficiencies in the system. That is our partnership. I know she trusts me to do that – we've both somehow shared something intimate.

(Field notes)

I was acutely aware that I had more opportunity for having a connected encounter with Louise than the midwives did whilst being a so-called non-participant in her care. This was a profound period for me in which I realised in a deep way that, as Leap (2000) states, 'The less we do, the more we give' (1). It also resonated with the phenomenological work of Bondas-Salonen (1998), who referred to women wanting midwives to be there and be mindful of the mother and the sense of isolation that an absence of this created.

As Louise (above) illustrated, women were subjected to not only routines and procedures but also an associated and profound sense of disconnection from midwives. In the rituals I observed and have described women were constrained by time: lack of time; fixing of time, both day and night; timing of bodily ministrations; and overriding of personal and bodily times with a rigid form of public time. In this way, women's bodies were disciplined as are those of prisoners or factory workers (Foucault 1977). As Frankenburg (1992b) states, 'The rigid time structures of the hospital emphasise the anti-temporality of the experience in relation to "normal" worldly time' (23). This anti-temporality was reinforced by a series of disconnected encounters that I now go on to discuss.

## Disconnected encounters

As already illustrated, communications on both sites appeared to be largely confined to what needed to be done. They were strikingly fragmented and disconnected from the woman's context, with little emphasis upon individual needs or concerns. This related in part to the impersonal nature of care, with midwives and women usually being complete strangers. The fragmented ways of working on both sites, combined with a rapid turnover of women, created very little continuity of carer and the midwives frequently commenced their working day being faced with having to relate to completely different women from those they related to on the previous day. The same applied to the women the midwives were attending to. The notion of developing any form of relationship with women was eerily absent. Under these circumstances, midwives were constrained from developing what Varcoe et al. (2003) refer to as an 'authentic presence' (966). To have presence is to 'come – unguarded, undistracted – and be fully present, fully engaged with whoever we are with' (Eldredge and Eldredge 2005: 138). Due to the constraints upon them, midwives tended to make rapid judgements about women that were not based on trusting relationships. Making rapid judgements inevitably led to labelling and stereotyping of women for the purposes of rapid action. This stereotyping, absence of relationality and lack of presence that I observed was strikingly resonant with that described by Kirkham and her colleagues (Kirkham 1999; Kirkham and Stapleton 2001b; Ball et al. 2002; Kirkham et al. 2002c).

A key way in which women's inner context was disregarded centred upon the lack of reference to women's birth experiences. There was little attempt to contextualise feeding with the earlier birth experience and in the time I was observing I saw only a few instances of midwives facilitating the mother in discussing her birth. Discussion around breastfeeding was rarely connected with women's previous feeding experiences, with other aspects of parenting, with women's lives or with their existing and personal knowledge. This can only be illustrated by an absence, rather than a presence, of quotes in which this connection took place. However, Barbara (P37) did go some way to highlight the disconnnectedness of encounters, 'I generally need more advice, but not necessarily breastfeeding, you know, knowing whether you've covered all the reasons why they get whingey, that sort of thing'. Stapleton *et al.* (2002c) also refer to the way in which midwives rarely explore women's existing personal knowledge and yet this is identified by women as important in relation to breastfeeding (Bowes and Domokos 1998; Whelan and Lupton 1998; Hoddinott and Pill 2000; Dykes 2003).

Being connected to networks of significant others has been shown to be important to new mothers (Bondas-Salonen 1998; Tarkka *et al.* 1998). However, the women I observed and interviewed not only experienced disconnected encounters with midwives but were commonly cut off from wider members of their social networks while in hospital. The need for women to draw upon others for information was rarely facilitated in the hospital setting, with placing in rooms designated for postnatal women, on both sites, being largely serendipitous. Sometimes a breastfeeding woman would be in a room on her own surrounded by women who were bottle feeding.

Barbara (P37), referred to above, was placed in a four-bedded bay with an antenatal woman and a multiparous mother who had changed from breastfeeding to bottle feeding. The other bed was empty for most of her stay. I observed her talking to this person; for example: 'He keeps putting his tongue up – I don't know what to do' and asking her questions such as, 'Am I better just ignoring him?' However, she got little in the way of an answer and as the other mother had stopped breastfeeding abruptly, her replies tended to be fairly negative. This absence of other mothers who were able to support a new breastfeeding mother made it difficult for the women to network and develop any sense of relationship with those surrounding them. This lack of emphasis upon creating a sense of community within the ward was highlighted by one of the midwives, Eunice:

> We don't do a baby bath demonstration any more, but when we did there was a lot of chit chat amongst the mothers and they used to ask a lot of questions. There isn't anywhere where we bring the mothers together now. The physio used to come and do exercises on the ward post-delivery and everyone used to do them together, but we don't bring anybody together at all now.
>
> (Eunice MW19)

One might expect that the day rooms would be places where women talked and networked with each other. However, the day room on one of the sites was very uninviting, and on the other site women could not take their babies into the day room because they were discouraged from walking around with their babies and wheeling the cot into the dayroom set off the security alarm.

On site two, network support was encouraged by an open visiting policy for partners. This appeared to be largely appreciated by women. Millie (P43) had her partner with her all of the time:

> He's going to stay here during the day, aren't you, while I try and have a sleep and see if she settles and then he can just see to her until she needs

another feed, until she won't settle anymore. Yesterday I was really tired after the night before and he came at nine in the morning and he just took her off me while I just got myself ready and had half an hours sleep, you know when she didn't need feeding, when she was just awake ... But ... um ... then when she was sleeping I got some sleep and then every time she made a noise I knew he was there to like see to her and check if she needed feeding, so I could concentrate on getting a little bit of sleep. So it's definitely a good idea, otherwise I'd be on my own all day [...]. He stays until about half eight when the visitors go of an evening, then I settle her down for the night and give her a bath.

(Millie, P43)

However, some partners were not necessarily particularly helpful in relation to women breastfeeding, being more anxious than their partners and leading to lowering of confidence in women. In some situations the partner appeared to dominate the woman rather than support her. Women tended to value advice from their mothers:

F: Has anyone talked with you about expression?
*Harriet (P52):* Not here, but my Mum went through quite a few things with me.
F: Oh, yes, you said she breastfed you.

However, women's mothers were often there amidst several other visitors, making mother-to-daughter encounters difficult. The disconnected encounters discussed here resonate with Kirkham's (1989) reference to 'linguistic non-touch technique', i.e. midwives not coming into 'contact with the woman's worries or concerns' (125–126). More than a decade later, Kirkham and Stapleton (2001a) highlight numerous further examples of this approach. The data I have presented here resonates with Fenwick *et al.*'s (2000, 2001) inhibitive nursing actions. Disconnected encounters were further exemplified and potentiated through the managerial approaches I observed and now describe.

### Managing breastfeeding

In Chapter 4 I discussed the ways in which women felt that they came under surveillance, creating feelings of being productive yet subjected. I now focus further upon the way in which encounters between midwives and mothers and the knowledge forms that midwives draw upon construct a situation in which women feel watched but strangely invisible, managed but not supported, told but not guided. The instrumental, managerial and authoritative approach adopted by midwives related to the requirements of the organisation, breastfeeding 'rules' and in some cases their lack of confidence in the bodily process of breastfeeding. As Shildrick (1997) states:

The objectifying gaze of the human sciences which fragments and divides the body against itself has its counterpart in an insight which equally finds the body untrustworthy and in need of governance. Moreover, each form of surveillance incites the other.

(55)

The organising theme of 'managing breastfeeding' illustrates an approach that disregards the woman and her personal agenda. The ritualistic management of 'breasts' and breastfeeding that I observed appeared to result in disembodiment and fragmentation of women's bodies. Shildrick (1997) refers to this destruction of the wholeness of 'one's being-in-the-world' as intrinsically compromising of 'feminine ontology'. The reproductive organs are referred to as discrete entities to be managed. 'The woman as a person plays little or no part, but is obscured as an intentional agent by the clinical concentration on a set of functional norms.' The woman's body is seen as a 'container' or 'bounded space' within which specific processes occur (Shildrick 1997: 25). The overriding of women's bodily boundaries that I repeatedly observed appeared to compound the sense for women that they were disconnected from their bodies and breasts.

The midwives tended to use reductionist language that suggested that they viewed breastfeeding as one component in a series of technical activities. The instrumental and goal-orientated philosophy thus objectified the woman's breast and rendered her as almost invisible. Many of the encounters between mothers and midwives related to breastfeeding centred upon the best ways to ensure the effective transfer of milk from mother to baby. Particular emphasis was placed on 'latching on,' more recently referred to as 'attachment'. This was also a major preoccupation for women as they commenced breastfeeding.

The emphasis upon this aspect of breastfeeding 'management' has grown considerably, related to research which links effective attachment to the mother's breast with improved breastfeeding outcomes; for example duration for which women breastfeed, reduction of sore nipples, and growth of the baby (Woolridge 1986a, 1986b; Righard and Alade 1992; Woods et al. 2002; Ingram et al. 2002). While this knowledge has undoubtedly brought gains for women in establishing effective breastfeeding, it has the potential to disrupt women's experiences when presented in a monologic, managerial way. Teaching technique has become supervalued over other ways of supporting women, leading to a technically prescriptive approach to care (Colson 1998a, 1998b). While rituals centring on rigid timing of feeds are fading, new rituals based on technical mastery and transfer of milk are appearing.

In my position as observer of practice during this study, I was very challenged by the emphasis upon technique. I am aware that there are indeed fundamental principles related to ensuring that breastfeeding is an effective process for the reasons stated above, but I did not wish to place myself in a position in which I was making positivistic and deterministic assumptions about the correctness of 'technique'. However, being able to see what was actually happening has added a perspective to this research which is absent from much of the sociologically focused literature on breastfeeding.

In spite of the emphasis upon the 'correct' attachment of the baby to her/his mother's breast, this 'technique' was not always facilitated effectively. For example, a midwife would miss out key points, like making sure the baby's mouth was wide open and bringing the baby's chin into the mother's breast, while focusing on less important points. This meant that a technical approach to women was prevalent in relation to their breastfeeding and yet women were not always facilitated in achieving the 'technique' effectively! Second, the teaching of specific techniques in reductionist ways and the issuing of pre-defined packages of information bypassed other needs which women had. The shortage of time increased this imbalance. This emphasis upon technical correctness may be seen in the following encounters:

| | |
|---|---|
| *Shannon (MW6):* | *(returns ten minutes after physically attaching the baby for Jackie (P33))* Has he come off? |
| *Jackie:* | I don't think he needs feeding at the moment. |
| *Shannon:* | When you're feeding you need to sit up straight, otherwise you'll get a backache. I like the underarm hold, it's more comfortable for me and quite good for latching on. Anyway, I'll come back later and help you breastfeed. |

Shannon gave prescriptive advice, apparently according to her own preferences, without any accompanying support or guidance. In the next scenario, Di likewise issued prescriptive advice but also assisted with feeding. However, she selected a time to assist that did not fit with the baby's desire to feed. This was another aspect of managing feeding which was dictated by the needs of the organisation rather than the mother's or baby's needs:

| | |
|---|---|
| | *(Di (MW18) was passing. Veronica was sitting in the chair after her shower and the baby had just started crying in the cot)* |
| *Di:* | Shall we have a go at feeding him? |
| *Veronica (P27):* | Yes, all right |
| *Di:* | How do you want to feed him? Sat up? |
| *Veronica:* | Yes, I think so ... |
| *Di:* | He's a big baby. Now then, when you're sitting you can try him across your lap or under your arm. Let's try this underarm position. OK, guide him with your hand. *(She guided Veronica's hands.)* Oh he's too angry to go on really. Let's try and wrap him up. *(Wrapped him up and tried again in underarm hold.)* Nipple upward towards the roof of his mouth. |
| | *(The baby latched on. The midwife sat with Veronica. The baby had a few suckles and then came off.)* |
| *Veronica:* | He's not really bothered now is he? |

| Di: | He's probably just wanting to be next to you. Shall we take him for his bath then? |
|---|---|
| Veronica: | Yes, I'll come too |
| Di: | You want to come do you? ... OK. |
| | *(Midwife and mother went to give the baby a bath.)* |

'Correct' or 'incorrect' technique was implied in one of the practices that I repeatedly saw. This involved the midwife approaching the woman, peering at the baby whilst feeding, making a cursory comment that the baby was on well and then leaving.

| Corinne (P41): | He's feeding all the time |
|---|---|
| Francesca (MW 28): | Frequent feeding is normal in the early days. *(Looked over at the baby feeding.)* He's on properly. |

The lack of clarification as to what 'being on properly' meant was highlighted by Barbara (P37): 'They've checked that he's on right, but I haven't really had a conversation about it'. Midwives rarely sat with a woman while she fed, to observe part or all of a breastfeed. Therefore, they would only get a snapshot and gained little sense of the dynamics of the feed and yet they made statements about the 'correctness' of the attachment with considerable authority. As I was in a position to observe breastfeeding for longer, I felt that the assessments of midwives were sometimes inadequate and women were not always feeding their babies in effective ways that would minimise nipple soreness.

Midwives often appeared to control interactions in accordance with their own pre-set agenda, providing information and assistance that they considered to be important and appropriate for women to receive. They largely appeared to ignore the woman's expressions of need for information in other areas, findings resonant with Kirkham *et al.* (2002a) and Stapleton *et al.* (2002b, 2002c, 2002d). An example of an encounter in which the midwife clearly had a pre-set agenda that differed to that of the woman illustrates this:

| Alex (MW9): | Would you like me to show you how to hand express? |
|---|---|
| Louise (P14): | No thanks, I don't really want to. |
| Alex: | Well it would reassure you that you have milk. |
| Louise: | Oh I can see that when she feeds. |
| Alex: | It's a technique we like to teach ladies. I'll just show you. |
| | *(She demonstrated on herself while Louise graciously listened, in spite of saying she was not interested. Done and ticked off!)* |

Louise discussed her feelings related to this afterwards:

> I wasn't ready for her telling me how to express. I wasn't at the stage where I wanted to know about that. I felt that things were going well and she was

latching on really well and I didn't see the need for expressing and I thought, 'well, she was determined to tell me'. She was trying to be helpful, but I was saying 'no it's all right I'm OK'. I knew that everything was all right because milk came out when she came off. I just think she wasn't listening to what I had to say. I think she thought she was doing me a favour, but I didn't want to know. I thought, 'well, if I need to know I'll ask you then'. I think they feel they have got to tell you certain things.

(Louise, P14)

Other participants echoed the sense that the midwife was not listening to their concerns; for example:

It would be nice if somebody could just come and spend ten minutes with you to talk about breastfeeding. If they did that they could learn about your concerns and anything you feel you need help with. I mean I'm not very confident at all *(laughs)*.

(Helen, P35)

In some cases midwives overrode women's concerns with unhelpful chatter:

*(Joy (MW4) passed the bed.)*

Grace (P28): He seems to go blue when he feeds.

Joy: Put him over your shoulder then. *(Took the baby from the mother and sat and winded him.)* Breastfed babies don't get much wind. Look at your lovely flowers. Beautiful aren't they? Is your other child a boy or a girl?

Grace: A boy.

Joy: Oh they're very different aren't they? No matter what people say, they are different. Men, I don't know why we bother with them *(laughs)*.

The midwife here completely led the agenda while the mother had no say in the course of the conversation. This is an example of the blocking of conversations, described by Kirkham (1989), in which questions were not answered properly and the conversation was diverted away from the subject about which women sought information. Fenwick *et al.* (2001) refer to the controlling nature of this form of 'dismissive chatter' which prevents or limits disclosure or depth of conversation (591).

The ways in which midwives conformed to an agenda that was not necessarily aligned to the women's resonates with the findings of others (Bondas-Salonen 1998; Levy 1999a, 1999b, 1999d; Lock 1999; Edwards 2000, 2005; Hoddinott and Pill 2000; Kirkham and Stapleton 2001a; Stapleton and Thomas 2001; Hunter 2002; Stapleton *et al.* 2002b). The reluctance I observed in women to interrupt the flow of the midwife's conversation was also reported by Stapleton *et al.* (2002c).

The resulting conversational dominance and asymmetrical style of interactions, with midwives taking control of the start of, the course of, and completion of interactions, has also been highlighted (Lomax and Robinson 1996; Lomax and Casey 1998; Stapleton *et al.* 2002b).

Unhelpful reference to personal experiences formed another way in which women's agendas were overridden. For example, in the following encounter Holly (MW7) approached Barbara (P37) who was struggling to settle her baby in the cot. She picked up the baby and stated, 'When I had my first baby I was ready for giving up – I said 'I'm tired and my boobs are hurting', but once I got home she was fine' (MW7).

Stella had been exposed to a midwife's personal problems and this led to her using nipple shields.

> I've got these nipple shields. My husband went and got them for me. When I was having Katie I was talking to one of the midwives and she'd had the same problem with her two children. She said with the last one even though they weren't miracle cures, they helped her carry on for a little bit longer, you know than she did with the first one. So [*partner's name*] went and got me some and I've used them this morning and yesterday. The lady came and showed me how to put them on. She suckles fine on them, but I just don't think she gets the same amount out as she would normally.
>
> (Stella, P46)

There were only a few examples of use of self, as midwives tended to adopt a formal approach to women. However, when midwives did use personal, experiential and embodied knowledge, it tended to be inappropriate. The inappropriate use of self is referred to by Battersby (2002), in a study centring upon midwives' attitudes to breastfeeding. This, she argues, relates to the need for midwives to experience some form of debriefing of personal experience during their undergraduate training. The notion of debriefing is central within the voluntary breastfeeding organisations and this reduces emotional residues stemming from unresolved breastfeeding issues. This makes way for congruence and appropriate use of self when considered to be helpful to a particular woman's situation (Smale, personal communication).

Women's boundaries were regularly eroded through being handled by midwives. I watched women's breastfeeding being managed and controlled, with midwives handling women's breasts in order to 'latch the baby on', often without seeking permission. This management and objectification of women's bodies undermined women's sense of confidence in that they were unable to repeat the actions themselves, requiring them to request help on several occasions during the course of a feed. This meant that their sense of dependency and inadequacy was reinforced and that they were susceptible to the combination of feelings of being almost separate from their bodies and breasts and yet enormously accountable for producing milk in appropriate amounts.

I was surprised that midwives appeared to be unaware that this 'hands-on approach' might be unacceptable to women. There is a growing literature now, based on women's negative comments about their breasts being handled, the baby being 'rammed' on to their breast and their desire to be taught breastfeeding skills verbally (Whelan and Lupton 1998; Vogel and Mitchell 1998; Mozingo *et al.* 2000; Hoddinott and Pill 2000; Ingram *et al.* 2002). However, to achieve this, midwives must be able to verbally articulate the skills required (Cox and Turnbull 1998; Vogel and Mitchell 1998; Whelan and Lupton 1998; Fletcher and Harris 2000; UNICEF UK 2001; Ingram *et al.* 2002). By sensitively articulating, rather than 'doing for' women, midwives may provide care which 'counteracts' rather than 're-enacts' earlier violations of women's bodies (Kitzinger 1992: 221).

Women who were post-Caesarean were particularly vulnerable to handling; for example Virginia (MW20) with Sue (P29) following her Caesarean section:

*Virginia (MW20):* Is your baby wanting a feed?

*Sue (P29):* Yes, but I can't feed like this, I think I need to sit up.

*Virginia:* I'll just call another midwife. *(The other midwife arrived and they sat her up in a semi-recumbent position which was not a helpful position for attaching the baby.)* Now then – *(The midwife, Virginia, took hold of the mother's breast and the baby and then whilst trying to 'connect' the two said):* do you mind if I help?

*Sue:* No

*Virginia:* He gets on but then he keeps slipping off. *(She turned to the student midwife.)* He needs to be close to mum, facing her and at the right height – there he's sucking nicely. The bottom lip should be turned down and the brown areola goes in and out if he's suckling well. They don't breastfeed all the time, they stop and start – that's normal.

*(She then turned to Sue):* All right I'll leave you for a little while.

*(Then to the student):* would you sit with her for a little while?

Women seemed to see the handling of their breasts following a Caesarean section as inevitable during the early stages. However, they expected this to be short-lived; for example:

*Sandra (P34):* Yesterday afternoon, the lady that was on, she did a lot of helping, trying to latch him on. They've all helped today. I wouldn't say advice, they've just helped trying to get him on, then they disappear off and he comes off again *(laughs)*. It's a lot easier when you've got two hands, to put your nipple into his mouth, but when you've got one hand and you're trying to do it yourself *(laughs)*.

| F: | So how do you feel about that type of assistance? |
|---|---|
| Sandra: | All right, I like them to help me, I mean at first, then once he gets used to latching on it should gradually get easier for me. |

This seen need for midwives to 'do for them' is referred to by Fleming (1998b) as 'supplementing' (141). In some cases a midwife would attach a baby for a mother and this would be accompanied by the sort of banter reminiscent of exhortations to the woman to push during labour, for example:

| Virginia (MW20): | What have you got at home? |
|---|---|
| Sue (P29): | Two boys. |
| Virginia: | Ooh, Two boys *(laughs)*. Well, what do you think. We'd better put him back on the breast, what do you think? Hungry Horace. We're going to have to put him back on; let's try the other side. |
| Sue: | All right. |
| | *(Midwife assisted her by holding the baby and mother's breast):* Um come on – *continued trying.* I'll just get you a pillow to bring him up a bit. |
| Sue: | I'd rather sit up a bit. |
| Virginia: | All right. *(She helped her to sit up.) (She tried again)* ... shhh; Mum's not very mobile at the moment is she *(laughs). (She continued trying.)* You're not taking a big mouthful at the moment are you ... oh come on. *(She said to Sue):* There's plenty there, you've got plenty of colostrum. |
| Sue: | He seems to give it a good suck and then pulls his head away. |
| Virginia: | We're trying to do it for you aren't we *(apologetically)*. Right go on, keep going ... Every which way but ... You're being silly, come on you're messing ... come on you're being silly ... Oh he's grabbed it there. *(The baby latched on)* ... ooh you're nicer than David Beckham, nicer than David Beckham aren't you ... come on. *(The baby continues to suckle)* ... Do you want me to leave the curtains around or not? |
| Sue: | No, I'm quite warm. |
| Virginia: | It is warm isn't it? *(She turned to me):* We're back on the breast again, it's going to be full time I think. *(She turned to the mother):* Still once things kick in and your lactation is going you'll be away won't you. *(She drew the curtain around.)* |
| Virginia: | *(to me, after she'd left Sue)* I think this one's going to need a lot of feeding! |

Some women actually used words such as 'being handled' and even 'mauled at': 'They manually help you' (Denise, P4); 'I tried expressing, the midwives tried, they mauled at them, but nothing came ... I've had midwives squeezing my nips and nothing coming out (Anna, P1). Sophie's 'hands-on' experience was accompanied by advice on being more forceful!

Sophie (P61):    He wasn't latching on properly ... so one of the midwives come and said ... be a bit more forceful ... just so they latch on a bit harder ... she did it herself just to show me and then I did it after ... so ... yeah ... but I don't know ... to me he's not over keen on it ... but I'll keep trying it and see how it goes.

F:    Mmm, so what have you learnt about latching on then?

Sophie:    Just be a bit more forceful than I was being ... I thought he was latched on when he wasn't ... you can tell ... it's a lot stronger ... (laughs) ... you can tell.

F:    I see ... so what do you mean by being a bit more forceful?

Sophie:    Just when they open the ... mouth ... to push it in ... just try it and push it in a little bit so that they do latch on (mimes an open mouth moving forward) ... instead of just latching on to the end and I could tell the difference when she showed me ... so he did better at half past six ... so we'll see on the next one (laughs).

Women's breasts were sometimes squeezed to 'reassure' women that they had enough milk: 'I've just said to the midwife I don't think I've got any milk and she said that I had and squeezed my nipple – and said look there's milk there' (Sam, P19).

Sam appeared to find the midwives' interventions helpful although it didn't seem to be assisting with confidence-building, 'The midwives are very helpful, doing it for me, because I'm not convinced I'm doing it right myself, so that I know I'm doing it right, they'll check it for me' (Sam, P19).

Some midwives assisted the women to hand express in order to give the milk by a cup to a baby having feeding problems. Again, the midwife sometimes carried this out with little in the way of explanation. Bryony (P7) was approached by the midwife who expressed her breast milk into a cup, without requesting permission, and with little explanation. She commented, 'they tell you to express but they don't actually show you how to do it' (Bryony, P7).

Smale (2000) highlights the need for awareness in health professionals that breasts are attached to real people, recognising the tensions inherent in relation to their advice, cultural norms and women's body image. Otherwise, she asserts, they may come to be seen as the 'nipple police' (2). Midwives not only unnecessarily breached women's bodily boundaries but also invaded women's wider spatial boundaries:

Shannon (MW6):    Right are you ready for feeding, love. (The baby was crying and mother was preparing to feed, sitting in the chair.)

Jackie (P33):    Yes.

| | |
|---|---|
| *Shannon:* | Right, I need you to get some of these teddies and things taken home cos we need some space, all right love? *(Established territory.)* |
| *Jackie:* | Yes, all right, I'll tell my husband this afternoon. |
| *Shannon:* | Let's get baby feeding under your arm. *(This midwife's preference from other observations.) (She moved forward and grasped the woman's breast and baby and put them together.)* All right, love we'll leave you to it. *(The baby came off in a couple of minutes. The mother looked tearful and carried on trying.)* |

This midwife firstly asserted her power in terms of what was 'allowed' in the space and then invaded the mother's bodily boundaries in her handling of her breast, without permission or discussion. I saw other examples of invasion of boundaries when midwives simply picked up babies without permission or discussion. I now discuss the ways in which midwives rationed information.

### Rationing information

Provision of information is of little use unless it is enabling or educationally useful. Women generally felt that they needed information from midwives. However, this was often delivered rapidly and with little reference to prior knowledge and understanding. The amount of information was commonly insufficient; in some cases it conflicted with other sources and in other situations it constituted misinformation. In some situations, the information being given was potentially detrimental to the establishment of an effective breastfeeding experience, although the women were often unaware of this.

The sense of temporal pressure upon midwives impacted on the ways in which they 'delivered' information, with speed being the essence as referred to by Jane (P12): 'The nurses are very good; they tell you everything very quickly, so sometimes it's like you've got to pick up everything very quickly, they're very quick ... but thorough.' As in Kirkham's (1989) labour ward study, the pressure on midwives' time led to 'information being compressed into dense routine packages' (127). This meant that women often felt that they had insufficient information to enable them to breastfeed effectively and with confidence. Veronica (P27) had stopped breastfeeding very early last time due to a feeling that she had insufficient milk and 'couldn't do it'. She felt that she needed more help this time:

| | |
|---|---|
| *Veronica (P27):* | I'm not too confident at the minute. I need more help with what to do, what positions to have him in, comfortable positions. |
| *F:* | Have you read about some of that or had some information about it? |
| *Veronica:* | I've read about it in a leaflet somewhere. *(Looks around at the locker.)* But nobody actually went through it with me this time. I |

> think they thought, 'well, you've had a baby before', they assume you know, you've been through it before.
>
> *F:* Would you have liked somebody to have gone through it with you?
>
> *Veronica:* Yeah, or asked me how I wanted to feed the baby. They didn't this time.

Women generally felt that they needed a more skills-based approach to teaching; for example:

> I'd like to be given help with the practical skills. You can read as much as you like but it needs to be more skill-based ... There seems to be a lack of information about breastfeeding.
>
> (Helen, P35)

This desire for more information related to practical skills required resonates with other studies; for example Britton (1998) and Hoddinott and Pill (1999a, 1999b). Some women received very little information from midwives about aspects of feeding, as illustrated in my interview with Tracy:

> *Tracy (P44):* I fed her just before I came on here *[postnatal ward]*. She was mooching round again *(turned her head to mimic rooting),* so I fed her, not very much because we had to come back up. Then she fed again this morning. I did it myself, but the nurse just came in and I asked her to check.
>
> *F:* Did you buzz her?
>
> *Tracy:* No she was around. She just popped her head in and said 'are you OK?', and I just asked her to check and she just said she's your baby, feed her when you want to feed her and she said you ask us if you're not sure about anything, ask us, but if you want to feed her whenever you like that's fine, and if you want any help just ask us. I mean I feel awkward about holding her, never mind breastfeeding her, but um ... I suppose that will come with time.
>
> *F:* Have you had any leaflets?
>
> *Tracy:* No ... I haven't.

From Tracy's account the encounters seem to have been dismissive and definitely did not meet her need for information. As referred to above, the information women gained tended to relate to how articulate they were in expressing their needs in this area and to how assertive they were in gaining access to a midwife's time. This inevitably disadvantaged women from lower socio-economic occupational groups, as highlighted by others (Bowes and Domokos 1998; Kirkham and Stapleton 2001b; Kirkham *et al.* 2002b).

On both sites, postnatal women were issued with a pack containing leaflets upon discharge, with those who were breastfeeding receiving some specific information on breastfeeding and those bottle feeding receiving specific information on making up bottle feeds. These leaflets were designed to be issued earlier as a part of the information-giving while women were on the ward, but I only saw this happen on a few occasions. I only saw one example of leaflets being referred to during a discussion of breastfeeding or being used to reinforce information given. Thus women were telling me they wanted more information but were usually unaware that these leaflets were available to them.

In some cases the leaflets were offered instead of giving information; for example:

Selina (P48):     Do you think I need to draw this nipple out with a niplette?
Felix (MW29):   Um, have you got the breastfeeding leaflet?
Selina:              Yes.
Felix:               Well, it tells you about hand expression on there. You could do that to draw your nipple out.

The only time the midwives appeared to make reference to the leaflet was as part of a very standard and monologic discharge 'patter'; for example Anthea (MW25) discussed the mother's haemoglobin level, her medication, six-week postnatal check, registration of the baby's birth, the leaflet about reducing the risk of sudden infant death syndrome, contraception, family planning clinics and the midwife's visit the next day. She then referred to the breastfeeding leaflet:

Anthea (MW25): Here's your breastfeeding leaflet 'Breastfeeding Your Baby'.
Annie (P42):      Yeah, thanks.
Anthea:             It shows you all the different ways of holding your baby and putting the baby on. Then there are some tips for breastfeeding. You might notice at about two to three weeks a slight milk reduction. It usually happens when you start to do a bit more. I'm mentioning it so that you won't need to worry if it happens. It may last for about twenty-four hours. It also tells you about expressing your milk and how to encourage your milk flow by gently kneading your breast to get your milk flowing. It also mentions breast pumps in here. Then there are these breastfeeding contact numbers here, so if you want any extra support you can ring one of these or you can ring your midwife and have a chat with her.
Annie:              Yeah, OK.
Anthea:             (goes through the postnatal discharge records) These are your exercises, and this is a leaflet about sterilisation and making up bottles which I'm sure you won't need to but just in case.

> There's a breastfeeding survey, so the Midwife will tick off how
> you are feeding at ten days.
>
> *Annie:* OK.

I heard this monologue several times and was amazed at its conformity within
and across midwives. The telephone numbers of follow-up breastfeeding supporters were supplied with the discharge pack but were rarely emphasised to
women. This data on leaflet use conforms to the findings of Kirkham and colleagues (Kirkham and Stapleton 2001a, 2001b; Stapleton *et al.* 2002a). Their
multi-methods study incorporated an ethnographic component involving observation and interviews to examine the use of evidence-based leaflets on informed
choice in maternity services. They concluded that while health professionals
were positive about the leaflets as a means to facilitate informed choices, competing demands within the clinical environment including time pressures
hindered and undermined their effective use. Midwives rarely held open discussions on the content of the leaflets. The leaflets themselves were rendered largely
invisible as they were commonly inserted into other leaflets, information or
hand-held notes.

The monologic nature of information-giving and absence of listening to
women meant that there was little attempt to elicit understanding; for example:

*Kerry (MW11):* Now breastfeeding ... has he had a feed?
*Laura (P16):* Yes, he fed once.
*Kerry:* Did he get on properly?
*Laura:* I think so.
*Kerry:* Right.

Women were commonly left in a rather confused state of mind regarding what
constituted effective feeding. I asked some of the women who had been given
some guidance on breastfeeding about the key principles associated with effective
breastfeeding. Frequently, the answers suggested that they had little understanding related to effective breastfeeding or the principles underpinning it:

*Mandy (P25):* The first night the midwives pointed out the principles.
*F:* Could you tell me what they are?
*Mandy:* Well, you guide the nipple around until he takes it, then you feel a
harder sensation. They told me about the ear movements.
*F:* Did they say anything about where to direct your nipple?
*Mandy:* Um, no not really.
*F:* How have you positioned yourself and him?
*Mandy:* Oh it's trial and error really, I've fed on my side mostly. *(The baby
was feeding on the side – not in a position that would facilitate
effective suckling.)*

*Chris (P32):*     She's on properly now, she's latched on properly, so hopefully, it should go right soon.

*F:*     So what do you mean by latching on properly?

*Chris:*     Um, trying to get all the nipple into her mouth so that she's like sucking most of it in her mouth, so she's not chewing on the end of the nipple ... then she doesn't get fed properly.

Conflicting information and/or advice is repeatedly referred to in relation to hospital practices and, as Krogstad *et al.* (2002) reflect, it often relates to a lack of a common approach, co-ordination and co-operation among health professionals. Conflicting information appears to be a continuing problem that undermines women's confidence in relation to breastfeeding, (Rajan 1993; Ball 1994; Garcia *et al.* 1998; Tarkka *et al.* 1998; Vogel and Mitchell 1998; Dykes and Williams 1999; Lavender *et al.* 2000; Simmons 2002a, 2002b). In this study, I saw a number of examples of conflicting information related to breastfeeding that stemmed in part from the attitude adopted by individual midwives. The problem of conflicting information and advice was then compounded by the lack of continuity of carer: 'Like I've seen different people this morning and they've all had a different approach' (Kate P39). Barbara (P37) expressed her distress:

> All he wants to do is just be on the breast. It's a bit tiring to be honest. I don't want that, but I must admit, I've had one nurse who said it's OK and one who said not to encourage it, so I am a bit ... do I or don't I ... sort of thing ... Because I don't particularly want to get into it, but I've been told it's OK, until your milk comes through ...
>
> (Barbara, P37)

Bryony (P7) appeared to passively accept a range of confusing and conflicting advice. However, when I asked her how she felt about her support she expressed deep dissatisfaction:

> I'm glad you are asking me about this because ... um ... I was going to write to someone about it. There are just so many people ... um ... there isn't a consistent game plan ... I find it all so confusing. They tell you to, um ... express but they don't actually show you how to do it. The midwife who saw me yesterday didn't have time to show me; she was in a rush. Anyway, you don't get the follow through. They are all helping but in different ways. It leaves me feeling guilty at not following advice ... um ... a team front is needed. They should be presenting one approach. There should be a leaflet on the problems too ... that would be useful.
>
> (Bryony, P7)

She saw the conflict as a form of politics. 'There's a lot of politics here between staff and I'm caught up in it. I shouldn't have to be in the middle of this.' She eloquently highlighted two philosophies of care, the time-driven mechanistic approach and a more sensitive closeness approach: 'There seem to be two schools of thought. The pumping and nipple shield and the hand expression and cup feed. The pumping ones seem to stress time shortage' (Bryony, P7).

While observing this mother I became acutely aware of her desire to avoid tensions in the relationships upon which she was dependent and her uncertainty as to how to socially negotiate encounters with midwives. These findings are supported by Hunt and Symonds (1995), Smale (1996), Bowes and Domokos (1998), Edwards (2000, 2005) and Curtis *et al.* (2001).

In some situations the advice given was simply misleading and counterproductive to effective feeding; for example Carol (P31) was told that she had sore nipples because she was 'freckly'. Amina (P23) expressed concern about her milk, to which the midwife both blocked her concern and gave some misleading advice:

*Amina (P23):*    I don't know if there's any milk?
*Charis (MW16):*    Just feed one side this time and one next time (subject changed).

Some women had adopted practices based on what appeared to be information that was confusing and therefore constituted misinformation. Millie was feeding from one side only, so that she was not stimulating her other breast at all:

*Millie (P43):*    She said try her out on different breasts if she wouldn't, you know, take from one, so I've only fed with one. I've fed her a couple of times, last night and she seems content with one.
*F:*    Did the midwives suggest you feed with one breast?
*Millie:*    Well, they actually told me that if she seemed content with the one just stick with the one for now and um, but if she's not taking to it I can change her over and see if there's any more milk in the other one, but up to now I've had enough in. I'm enjoying it though. It's definitely hard work, but um definitely worth it ... I think I should be able to manage it. I was speaking to the midwife and she was saying about like ... get some formula milk in just in case, should you ever run down and she's not feeding and you know your milk's not strong enough or whatever ... She said I'm not really supposed to say this but for your sake just get some in handy otherwise you're going to be too tired, but she said just persevere for as long as you can but for your sake just have some in handy and you don't have to use it if you don't want to ...

It is ironic that the midwife suggested that Millie buy some formula milk just in case. Indeed, if Millie continued to receive misinformation about breastfeeding this suggestion might become a self-fulfilling prophecy!

## Midwifery work: 'productive yet subjected'

I have highlighted key elements of encounters that constituted a 'failure to touch base' with women as they sought to grow in confidence with breastfeeding during the first days following the birth. These findings resonate strongly with the encounters described by Fenwick *et al.* (2000, 2001) as inhibitive nursing actions. The midwives, like the postnatal women, were 'productive' yet 'subjected'. They were heavily constrained by linear time, in that their work was unpredictable and rushed, coping with women who were usually complete or almost complete strangers. Their work was time pressured, routine, disconnected, fragmented and unsatisfying. In this context they saw themselves as 'supplying' a service under extremely 'demanding' conditions. By highlighting these constraints upon midwives within a medicalised, institutionalised culture, the postnatal ward, I add to the critical theory generated by Kirkham and colleagues (Kirkham 1999; Kirkham and Stapleton 2001b; Ball *et al.* 2002).

To support understanding of the ways in which midwives cope with these demands I have drawn upon the concept of emotion work (Hunter 2002, 2004, 2005). Like that of the mothers, midwives' work was conducted out of relationship or relational context and this meant that their actions were seen as 'one-way' and therefore emotionally draining. Midwives engaged in ways of coping (emotionally managing) with the pressure and chaos. This included adopting rituals and routines and approaching women in disconnected, monologic, directive and managerial ways. The focus appeared to be upon the needs of the institution first, with mothers and babies second, as described by others (Lock 1999; Hunter 2002, 2004, 2005; Deery 2003, 2005). Satisfaction was gained by completing tasks, ticking them off and writing up the paperwork.

There was a striking absence of reference to the women's personal embodied knowledge and experiences. The encounters were largely characterised by monologue and consequently overrode women's agendas and silenced them. The women were therefore subjected to an experience of breastfeeding a new baby in a public place, surrounded by strangers who adopted a largely instrumental and managerial approach. They had to constantly compete for a midwife's time and attention. This culture left women feeling physically 'managed' but emotionally vulnerable. It was counterproductive to the building of women's confidence and emotional recuperation. The atmosphere and encounters reinforced women's sense of alienation and separation from their body and appeared to inhibit development of relationality with their babies, as referred to by others (Lock 1999; Fenwick *et al.* 2000, 2001). However, there were some exceptions to the above in which midwives created situations for women to feel emotionally safe and to grow in confidence; I now turn to these.

## Taking time and 'touching base'

In this section I focus upon encounters that assisted women in coping with uncertainty, sensitively encouraged them to persevere, built their confidence and supported them in developing the practical skills to carry out breastfeeding effectively. In a country like the UK where the bottle of formula milk dominates, women have often had little in the way of previous positive personal experiences of successful breastfeeding and minimal exposure to others breastfeeding, particularly in socially deprived communities. This means that emotional, esteem, practical, informational and network support from health professionals becomes particularly important.

Professional encouragement and confidence-building appear repeatedly in the literature as important to breastfeeding women (Ball 1994; Schy *et al.* 1996; Humenick *et al.* 1998; Svedulf *et al.* 1998; Hoddinott and Pill 2000; Gill 2001; McCreath *et al.* 2001; Hauck *et al.* 2002; Ingram *et al.* 2002). Thus, encounters with what Bandura (1995) describes as self-efficacy (self-confidence) builders would appear to be crucial for women, especially during the most vulnerable first days. Bandura (1995) highlights some of the characteristics of self-efficacy builders; for example 'raising people's beliefs in their capabilities', structuring situations for them 'in ways that bring success and avoid placing people in situations prematurely where they are likely to fail often [...]. They encourage individuals to measure their success in terms of self-improvement rather than by triumph over others' (4). Thus they convey validation and positive appraisals, creating situations in which people can achieve success, 'modelling for others how to manage difficult situations', 'demonstrating the value of perseverance' and 'providing positive incentives and resources for efficacious coping' (10).

Davis-Floyd and St John (1998) employ the metaphor of the 'bridge' as a symbol representing physicians who had undergone a transformative journey from techno-medicine to holistic healing in their attempts to mediate between the paradigms (231). In a sense this was what I saw when I observed certain midwives attempting to provide a bridge between a clinical institution with its time-driven production-line ethos and the personal needs of individual women. In the case of the breastfeeding mother there was also a need to facilitate the women in feeling connected and in relationship with their babies, as emphasised by Fenwick *et al.* (2000, 2001).

There is a dearth of literature relating to the confidence-building role of the midwife in relation to breastfeeding women in hospital. As stated, research on professional assistance for breastfeeding women normally relates to components and timing of a 'package' of information; for example Righard and Alade (1992), Schy *et al.* (1996), Carson (2001), Woods *et al.* (2002). It has placed less emphasis on the types of encounter with midwives that women find enhance or undermine their confidence and contribute to whether they feel enabled or not to persevere with breastfeeding whilst in hospital.

Given the clinical culture in which the midwives were working, I became intrigued as to why some individuals were different in their approach. It became evident to me that these midwives had a profound belief in the value of supporting breastfeeding women. They demonstrated a determination to overcome temporal and relational barriers and this, in some cases, was combined with fewer external time/unpredictability constraints upon them and therefore a greater sense of temporal autonomy, even if transient. However, I am unable to record some of the comments made about the personal cost to them of 'swimming against the tide' as they wished this to remain 'off the record'.

I observed only a few examples of encounters in which midwives endeavoured to take time and touch base with women; indeed I had to actively search out midwives who worked differently (discrepant cases). It was quite difficult to break down the data on supportive encounters in that by its very nature such an interaction was helpful through its multifaceted and synergistic nature. Therefore, I present this data by referring to specific midwives and the ways in which their encounters were supportive to breastfeeding women.

### Tasmin: connecting

Tasmin was a mature midwife with a degree in midwifery. The day I saw her at her most enabling was when she had come to the ward from clinic because it was not busy. She was therefore just helping out with no sense of having to account for her 'output'. She appeared to listen to and learn from the mother and respond to her cues; for example during a postnatal examination:

| | |
|---|---|
| Tasmin (MW3): | How was your birth? |
| | *(Mother talked for a few minutes about her birth. Tasmin actively listened to her story.)* |
| Tasmin: | So have you any stitches? |
| Julie (P9): | No. |
| Tasmin: | That's good. |
| Julie: | But I've passed a clot. |
| | *(Tasmin and Julie discussed the size of the clot and Tasmin suggested that Julie show a midwife next time, if possible. Temperature (under arm) and blood pressure taken. A discussion continued about the birth while waiting for the thermometer. The mother was reassured that the readings are fine.)* |
| Tasmin: | How did you sleep? *(Short discussion took place about sleep, related to the birth again. Tasmin asked Julie about her other children.)* |
| Tasmin: | I'll just feel your tummy – your uterus is lovely and firm – would you like to feel it yourself? |
| Julie: | Oh yes – *(Tasmin guided her hand.)* |
| Tasmin: | How are your legs? *(Short discussion regarding cramp.)* |
| Tasmin: | Did you breastfeed your other children? |
| Julie: | No, this is the first time. |
| Tasmin: | How do your breasts feel? |
| Julie: | My nipples are a bit sore. He wants to have something in his mouth all the time. |

| | |
|---|---|
| *Tasmin:* | He needs to suckle as much as possible because that helps with your milk supply. At first it is colostrum which is very thick and very nutritious. Then your breasts will start to feel full in a day or two and the milk will change, then your breasts will become more comfy again. The milk at the start of the feed is called first milk and then it becomes richer so you need to leave him on for some time. I remember when I fed mine she seemed to like one side better than the other, but I thought it would have been the other side. |
| *Julie:* | Yes, I like my left breast best, but he seems to like my right. *(The mother became more animated by sharing of information.)* What can I put on my nipples to stop them cracking and that? |
| *Tasmin:* | Well, they may be uncomfortable the first couple of days, but if you get someone to check how he's on your breast then they should feel better. You can express a bit of milk and let air get to your breasts. Next time he wakes up we'll have a look. |
| *Julie:* | Will he need water? |
| *Tasmin:* | No, he doesn't need extra water. Remember as well that each baby is different and often they want to feed very frequently at first, but later they feed less frequently. |
| *Julie:* | How long did you feed yours? |
| *Tasmin:* | Oh until nine months. |
| *Julie:* | What about her teeth? |
| *Tasmin:* | Well somehow they don't seem to bite you when they have got teeth. |
| *Julie:* | Oh, because I was worried about that. |
| *Tasmin:* | And it's good to keep feeding, as it's so full of goodness. |
| *Julie:* | I've heard it reduces eczema? |
| *Tasmin:* | Yes, that's right, it's a good idea. Well he looks great, when he wakes up either I or the other midwife will check him as well. I'll just go and get your postnatal exercise leaflets. *(She came back and discussed postnatal exercises.)* |

This was an encounter in which the midwife and mother did not know each other and yet a rapport was built up quickly whereby the mother was able to explore a range of issues that were of concern to her. Tasmin contextualised breastfeeding with Julie's birth, asking her about her birth experience to which she actively listened. She then contextualised it with Julie's life by enquiring about her other children. The encounter illustrates information-giving in response to the mother's cues; for example 'He wants to have something in his mouth all the time'. The information was then given in a way to enhance the mother's understanding of the principles underpinning baby-led feeding. Tasmin also sensitively shared personal experiences. I rarely saw this use of self, probably due to the culture within which midwives were working in making them unable or unwilling to draw on and use their own experiential learning as mothers (Kirkham 1989).

The personal revelation offered by Tasmin, i.e. 'I remember when I fed mine she seemed to like one side better than the other, but I thought it would have been the other side', assisted the mother in relating to her and created an opening for her to ask questions: 'Yes, I like my left breast best, but he seems to like my right. What can I put on my nipples to stop them cracking and that?' A discussion followed about prevention of sore nipples. This use of personal experience in a sensitive way relates to that described by Fenwick *et al.* (2000, 2001). Tasmin also emphasised the individuality and uncertainty of feeding: 'Remember as well that each baby is different and often they want to feed very frequently at first, but later they feed less frequently.' I interviewed Julie (P9) following this encounter:

*F:*     Could I just ask you how you feel after the discussion you have just had with the midwife?

*Julie:*  Well it has stopped me panicking that he isn't getting enough because he is really.

*F:*     Yes, what has reassured you on that?

*Julie:*  Because the midwife breastfed herself, her own babies; she's not just saying it because she's read it, she's saying it because she knows.

*F:*     How does that reassure you?

*Julie:*  You know, she's not just got it out of a book and she's saying it. She obviously knows herself because she's done it three times – yeah. Everybody has been so negative, but it's not the case all the time.

*F:*     What else did you learn from the discussion?

*Julie:*  Well I don't need to give extra drinks, he doesn't need extra and she said I didn't need a dummy, it's just the baby building the supply up. I thought he was just stuck on it because he wanted a bit of comfort, see I didn't know that. I would have just stuck a dummy in his mouth. So now I'll persevere – I'll try not to give it. I don't feel disheartened now.

I had only a brief chance to ask Tasmin about the interaction because she had to return to clinic:

*F:*     I notice you share with women some of your own experiences as a mother?

*Tasmin:*  Oh, well, I share my experiences in response to intuitive cues. I'm very careful about how I do it. I wouldn't always do it, but I do it with sensitivity when I need to. I do it fairly spontaneously when I think it's relevant.

This was the only one of two references to midwives using intuitive cues made during the study which points to the general lack of acknowledgement of its relevance or even existence. Tasmin also demonstrated active listening, a key aspect of caring (Kirkham 1993; Bondas-Salonen 1998; Davis-Floyd and St. John 1998; Fenwick *et al.* 1999, 2000, 2001; Pairman 2000). Davis-Floyd and

St. John (1998) emphasise the importance of listening and sharing in recreating a place for the 'human values of partnership, relationship, compassion, and caring' (107). Kirkham (1993) states, 'we need to let women speak in order to know their concerns and to improve our ability to listen to women's words and cues' (9).

In order to see how Tasmin's approach may have changed on a very busy day when she was rushing from one person to another I actively sought to observe her during such times. She was asked by Kate (P39) to come and check her breast-feeding. She said to me, 'If you're observing this interaction, it's going to be VERY quick. I've got an antenatal woman with problems over the other side, so I've only got two minutes'. The encounter was therefore quite directive but she did get across some key points within a very short space of time:

*Tasmin:* Now lets see what I can do? Are you comfy? Lets take away these extra blankets ... that's better, now, aim to put her chest next to yours. Line her up nicely and point her nose to about level with your nipple. Then make sure her mouth is really wide open, yes ... tease her lips with your nipple, that's it; yes, good now bring her on quickly. *(Mother does this as Tasmin watches for a minute, then she apologises and goes. Her baby attaches well and suckles for a while.)*

I then asked Kate:

*F:* How do you feel after that time with the midwife?

*Kate (P39):* Well that's the first time I've been shown what to do. Now I understand what to do. I wish they'd told me that, you know, earlier and I wouldn't have needed to keep buzzing them.

This very brief encounter was 'good enough' (Allan 2000) under the circumstances and the mother was pleased to have been shown, albeit rapidly, how to attach her baby effectively. The encounter illustrates the way in which this midwife changed her approach given the constraints, but did what she felt was most effective. I would have liked to have observed her assisting a woman with attachment when there was more time, but did not get the opportunity as Tasmin was rarely on this ward as she tended to be one of the midwives who was frequently asked to go to delivery suite, clinic or theatre!

### Leanne: touching base

The contextualisation with the woman's birth and life and response to women's concerns was also evident in a dialogue between Leanne (MW17) and Sue (P29). Leanne also supported the mother sensitively through the process of breastfeeding and made time to stay with her for a while.

| | |
|---|---|
| *Leanne MW17):* | *(Introduced herself. The baby was crying)* How are you? |
| *Sue (P29):* | Oh, all right, but I can't move myself much. |
| *Leanne:* | How was your birth? |
| *Sue:* | Well, I ended up with a Caesarean because the cord came down. |
| *Leanne:* | Oh, did you have a general anaesthetic? |
| *Sue:* | Yeah, so I'm half asleep now and I can't move around much. |
| *Leanne:* | Mmm, you'll feel a lot better when you are more mobile. Let's see if we can help you? *(She stood by and encouraged Sue to support her baby.)* Can you support him yourself with your arm? |
| *Sue:* | Yeah |
| *Leanne:* | Good; now aim your breast up to the roof of his mouth – that's it; I'll just watch. *(Baby attached and suckling.)* Have you got other children? |
| *Sue:* | Yeah I've got two boys at home. |
| *Leanne:* | How did you feed them? |
| *Sue:* | I fed the first one for two weeks then I got mastitis and ended up giving up. Then the same thing happened again with my second one, but my community midwife was really helpful so I fed him for six months. That was three years ago. |
| *Leanne:* | That's good; you did well ... *(silence while she observed the feed).* They stop and start, so don't worry. Sometimes when you have a Caesarean section it takes a little longer for them to get going. You may find feeding on your side helpful and sometimes skin contact can be useful just to calm him. How does that feel? |
| *Sue:* | OK, but the after pains are awful. |
| *Leanne:* | Yes; they'll be stronger when you feed him at your breast, because it's helping your uterus to contract down ... You can see he's starting to take lovely deep sucks. So have your other children been in to see him? |
| *Sue:* | No they'll be in today. |
| *Leanne:* | Have you got a name for him? |
| *Sue:* | Yes [name]. |
| *Leanne:* | Do you feel you have enough knowledge about mastitis? |
| *Sue:* | Um, why do women get it? |
| *Leanne:* | It can be for various reasons, it could be poor drainage if the baby isn't well attached or isn't finishing the breast feed, or a tight fitting bra. The thing to do is to wait until the baby comes off your breast, try not to take him off before he's ready. I've got a very good leaflet on mastitis, I'll bring you a copy when I come back a little later. *(She did this later and talked her through it.)* |
| *Sue:* | Thanks. |

Leanne 'touched base' with Sue by asking about her birth, her other children and her current concerns. This enabled her to then provide useful information that focused upon individual needs and concerns; for example with regards to mastitis. This contrasted with the standard patter seen in many encounters. Leanne also used positive language to emphasise progress, 'You can see he's starting to take lovely deep sucks'.

### Jenny: taking time, establishing trust and building confidence

I shadowed Jenny (MW14) over a period of several days as she supported Jocelyn (P18) through her five-day postnatal stay. Jocelyn came from an area with high levels of social deprivation. She had two older children at home. Her current baby was born at thirty-six-plus weeks gestation and was also small for gestational age. Jenny touched base with Jocelyn in several ways, meeting her needs for emotional, esteem, informational and practical support. One example of confidence-building, an aspect of esteem support, may be seen in the following dialogue:

| | |
|---|---|
| *Jocelyn (P18):* | Is he feeding all right? |
| *Jenny (MW14):* | Your body feelings are the best guide. What do you think? |
| *Jocelyn:* | I can hear him sucking. |
| *Jenny:* | Yes and I can hear him swallowing. Oh look, you can see milk dribbling out on to his chin! That's good. |

Here Jenny assisted Jocelyn in connecting with her own embodied signals and confirmed these by way of reassuring her about the adequacy of her milk. This 'process of inspiring confidence in women by our confidence in their abilities' is referred to by Leap (2000: 7). Another key way in which Jenny built Jocelyn's confidence centred upon emphasising a sense of progress and achievement: 'Oh that's great! He's really suckling keenly there. He's really progressing.' One of the most striking observations I made when observing Jocelyn and Jenny was the way in which Jenny was there for Jocelyn, forming a relationship with her. This relationship was assisted by there being continuity of carer, but it was more than that. It was a relationship of trust. As stated, this ability to form a trusting relationship is now emerging in the literature as enormously beneficial to women and the quality of their maternity care experience (Halldorsdottir and Karlsdottir 1996a, 1996b; Edwards 2000, 2001, 2005; Fenwick *et al.* 2000, 2001; Pairman 2000; Curtis *et al.* 2001). As Edwards' (2000) research showed, 'where trust was the foundation of the relationship between the woman and her midwife, the woman interpreted her experience in terms of growth and change' (77). Jocelyn's trust in Jenny appeared to be fundamental to the incremental confidence-building that took place:

> I couldn't have done it without Jenny. She's been fantastic. She has been with me every day and has really helped me, building my confidence by praise and

saying, 'You're doing fine'. She was there regular like, you know, same midwife. She knew exactly what was going on. She spends time with you.

Following comments from Jocelyn that Jenny helped her to feel more confident, I asked Jenny how she had attempted to build her confidence:

Well I kept hammering away that it would get better, it would get easier and that baby was doing very well with that weight and with those problems. I got the feeling that eventually that was filtering through to her, but initially it was just running off her, you know she was just unsettled, insecure, wasn't even certain that she wanted to go on feeding ... and that was my conscious tactic anyway, you know, to keep bashing away and that it will be OK and that she was doing very well. It seemed to work. With all that's going on she's got a very poor attention span and there's a sort of low-grade chaos surrounding the whole thing. She was often ... she would start a conversation and then I noticed she veered off into the distance half way through. She seemed to find it quite taxing to get involved in a sort of planning discussion as to what to do with the next feed. Literally, I would see her just staring out of the window, just cutting off. Um, once I realised that, I tailored my approach towards her, to give less information and to keep the horizons down to the next hour or two rather than the long term.

(Jenny, MW14)

Here Jenny emphasises her growing understanding of Jocelyn's needs and her tailoring of information to meet her individual needs. She recognised that Jocelyn felt uncertain and unsure of herself and needed to be supported by discussion of short- rather than long-term issues at this stage. This understanding and tailoring of support could only occur in a situation in which the midwife and mother had time together to get to know each other. The way in which Jenny helped Jocelyn to cope in this context is summed up well by Leap (2000). She uses the metaphor of the journey, in which the terrain is rocky, as she emphasises the value of the midwife and mother 'embracing uncertainty together' (4):

The midwife provides a map for the woman if she needs one, warning her at the same time that the journey includes uncharted landscapes for which there can be no planning. She points out the sign posts for various alternative routes and warns of hazards to avoid or obstacles that can be circumvented or surmounted.

(Leap 2000: 15)

Jocelyn's emphasis upon time resonates with the findings of Curtis et al. (2001) who reported that maternity care service users described staff who 'made time for them' as giving 'good care' (128). However, Jenny pointed out that the opportunity to follow a woman through and develop a relationship was quite unique:

I've been involved with Jocelyn from transfer to this ward. It's one of those lovely situations where she's had the same person most of the time. I mean so often you see someone one day, you set things in motion and the next day someone else has scuppered it. The thing is; this is the exception. We've been quiet over the weekend. I've spent hours with her. Normally though, she just wouldn't have got anything like this attention and she would have ended up most probably with the baby in neonatal unit. She's got a poor ability to retain information and she just could not have coped with minimal attention. Then because of lack of staff she would have ended up separated from the baby and all that extra time and expense would be involved with a baby on neonatal unit. That is what happens when there aren't the staff. It's just been lovely to be able to support someone through this process like this.

When asked about how her care might have changed in a busier situation, Jenny stated:

Well, I think there's more pressure when you're busy not to discuss things and just to tell a mother what to do, and because most mothers, particularly in a stressed situation like that, will just do what you tell them it's very easy to fall into a situation where you almost exploit that. I mean given the current situation you cannot give woman-centred care. I mean I would hope I still discuss things with women and try to discuss things with them. But it's incredibly difficult with someone who's a bit slow, who needs time; time to burst into tears and then settle down afterwards.

To summarise, Jenny touched base with Jocelyn in several ways. She followed her through her hospital stay until discharge and she made considerable time for her. She built up a relationship of trust with Jocelyn and used an approach that was based upon understanding her as an individual. She made clear plans of support that were carefully communicated to the staff who came on at the next 'shift'. She built Jocelyn's confidence and she encouraged her to persevere, by providing small short-term goals. She helped her to cope with the uncertainty and emphasised progress being made. She encouraged Jocelyn to listen to intuitive cues, thus helping her to feel competent at making judgements herself.

The encounters between Jenny and Jocelyn, when compared with some of the interactions described above, illustrate that despite the organisational culture there are different styles of caring. Jenny's style was facilitative in contrast to more authoritative, directive and insensitive approaches of some of the midwives referred to earlier. This difference in approaches by individual midwives, ranging from unsupportive to supportive encounters, is described by others (Berg *et al.* 1996; Halldorsdottir and Karlsdottir 1996a, 1996b; Fenwick *et al.* 2000; Kirkham 2000a). Nevertheless, as Jenny highlights, the ability to support women in a facilitative way is hindered by organisational constraints.

Jenny had worked hard to create the relationship she knew would support, encourage and build Jocelyn's confidence and help her cope with her emotions. However, it was clear to me that providing this type of care left Jenny marginalised and isolated among the majority of the staff. She was working against the prevailing culture on the postnatal wards to form meaningful relationships based on trust and to provide a high level of support. The challenge of achieving this within institutionalised settings in which this form of care is not the norm is dramatically highlighted by a series of works by Kirkham and colleagues (Kirkham 1999, 2000a; Edwards 2000, 2005; Kirkham and Stapleton 2000; Kirkham and Stapleton 2001a; Ball *et al.* 2002; Stapleton *et al.* 2002a, 2002d, 2002e). As Fleming (1998a) states in relation to midwives who take the lead from how the woman feels:

> Midwives, in attempting to practise within a framework which is different from that of the dominant medical model of birth, and which is accepting of the women as a partner in her own experience, are basing their clinical judgement on knowledge which does not come from traditional Western epistemologies.
>
> (11)

In contrast, as Wilkins (2000) asserts, the western 'professional outlook' of midwifery has made it 'conceptually blind' to the processes that make a relationship 'special for mothers' (29).

### Kim: building networks

Kim was pregnant and worked part-time. She was 'not allowed' to be called to delivery suite due to being pregnant, so when she came onto the ward she therefore felt more secure. She appeared to connect with the women because she was pregnant. She shared of herself and women saw her pregnancy as an opening point for conversation. The encounters were non-directive and woman-centred. In the following extract from my field notes I illustrate how she created an atmosphere which assisted women in developing a network of support from other mothers:

> I observed Kim (MW15) during a morning. She was based in one bay where she largely stayed, focusing particularly on a woman who had just returned from having a Caesarean section under general anaesthetic and who needed a lot of assistance with breastfeeding. The woman spoke little English, so I didn't approach her. Kim was sensitively assisting the mother with breastfeeding, quietly observing the feed and also making herself available to the other women. The other three women were also breastfeeding. The three other women asked her questions about her forthcoming baby and her existing family, which she answered as a mother to mother. They also asked her

many questions of concern to them that she answered in a very non-directive and non-authoritative way drawing on her combined experience of being a mother and a midwife. She had a very facilitative style, drawing the mothers into the conversation. The women started to chat among themselves with increasing freedom and confidence both when she was there and when she wasn't. I observed a huge amount of exchange of useful discussion and suggestions related to breastfeeding and parenting in general, which was clearly the women's main concern at this point.

(Field notes)

This facilitation of what Leap (2000) describes as the fourth 'C' – 'Community' (8), involving encouraging the development of supportive relationships and enabling women to learn from each other, is commonly overlooked in hospital. The limited visiting hours often make it difficult for women to communicate effectively with their community network of social support. The system by which the women could only phone out using a portable phone that was often much in demand or out of order created a further barrier to communication with the outside world. The importance of psychosocial factors such as sensitive social support, particularly network support and social cohesion, upon health and well-being are clearly recognised (Sarafino 1994; Wilkinson 1996). Wilkinson (1996) argues that collectivism, sharing and reciprocity were cultural norms, globally, for most of human existence until the outset of capitalism and consumerism, bringing with them a philosophy of individualism.

The 'chatting' between Kim and the women in the bay was akin to that described by Fenwick et al. (2001). They describe this sharing generated by 'chatting' – i.e. relating, exchanging and sharing lifestyles. They refer to talking as changing the atmosphere. Yet in their study, only twelve per cent of communications at the bedside contained examples of chatting. The facilitative interaction was described as:

No one person appeared to be guiding the turn taking or setting the agenda. Women were 'noted' to be engaged in the conversation, asking questions of the nurse and leading the discussion. The nurse appeared comfortable in the exchange. Both participants shared equally and the interactions were characterised by a sense of equality.

(588)

They noted that self-disclosure by the nurses, through informal chatter, encouraged similar disclosure by the woman, enabling nurses to access the woman's world. They were sharing rather than telling. They noted that elements found in 'chat', including 'asserting similarity', 'displaying empathy', 'calming reciprocity' and using 'conversation politeness gestures', all enhanced the other's sense of self (590).

## Essences of taking time and touching base

In this section I have highlighted some of the ways in which midwives 'took time' and 'touched base', that is touched the personal experience of women and supported them in relation to breastfeeding their babies. The strategies utilised included contextualising breastfeeding with the woman's birth and personal experiences in general. There were examples of active listening, sensitive use of self and an individualised approach to care. Ways of building confidence included assisting women to connect with their own bodies and babies' signals, validating the women's experiences, encouraging and praising women, and emphasising progress and achievement. Women were supported with understanding the principles of effective feeding as appropriate to their situation. Midwives found ways of making enough time to meet the needs of the women. Opportunities to create networks with other women were created. Sadly, these examples were very few as relationships between mothers and midwives were almost impossible to establish and few of the midwives appeared to truly seek ways of working in connection with women or indeed even appeared to have the desire or ability to do this.

So how can we reconstruct a culture in which the concepts of embodiment, relational skill and caring/nurturance are celebrated and made possible in postnatal midwifery practice? How may the midwife–mother relationship be one that values connected encounters in which midwives touch base with women, meeting their individual needs in the context of their lives? How may we ensure a dramatic move away from an instrumental, technical and authoritative approach to breastfeeding women which causes them to feel that they are reduced to being productive yet subjected? To what extent can real change be achieved within a hospital-based maternity unit given the origins, nature and culture of hospital institutions? I now address these issues in Chapter 6.

# Breastfeeding and midwifery work

## Re-conceptualising bodies, time and relationships

People want everything in black and white ... but being a new mother and breastfeeding are not like that at all. Breastfeeding is like midwifery, you have to wait and see what happens, you don't know what is going to happen next. You have to go with the flow ... There's no answer to breastfeeding – it's complicated, people have different lives, different circumstances and different pressures from outside. I know that from my own experience of breastfeeding. Then midwives bring their own attitudes. It's very complex.

(Virginia, MW20)

## Introduction

In this chapter, I illustrate the striking parallels between breastfeeding women and midwives and assert that both are engaged in 'productive' activities under challenging conditions. 'Supplying' for another's needs in a culture that focuses upon 'racing against the clock' leads to both mothers and midwives constructing ways of coping and controlling. Given this scenario, I discuss implications for practice and policy. I make recommendations for a reconsideration of the way in which women's bodies are understood and experienced, a re-conceptualisation of women's time, reconfiguration of knowledge about breastfeeding, re-visioning of the mother–baby and midwife–mother relationships and relocation of the place and space in which mothers commence their breastfeeding journey.

The experience for the women is encapsulated by the metaphor of the production line and its accompanying notions of efficient production and supply against linear time, with all of the associated demands upon those engaged in the production process. The postnatal ward was the final hospital stop of a medicalised journey in which women's bodies were subjected to multiple measures and timings of the quality and pace of their productivity. On the postnatal ward women entered a place in which they were engaged in a new form of productivity involving the making and delivering of their breast milk to their young baby. This was a part of the project of motherhood to produce a new citizen who could meet the needs of society.

Women conceptualised their bodies as vessels that were apart from them and functioning (or not) despite them. There was a sense of alienation and separation from the product, breast milk. These dualistic understandings of their bodies were reinforced within the hospital setting through the mechanistic monologues of midwives. Women's productive projects were largely viewed by the women themselves as transient and temporary as they planned, even at this early stage, for their return to their 'normal' productive lives with return to paid employment being a central consideration.

Women's productive projects involved supplying milk and meeting their baby's demands. However, almost without exception, women expressed doubts about their bodies' ability to supply. The exceptions were among those who had previously breastfed and for whom the experience had been a positive one. Women reflected a deep mistrust in the efficacy of their bodies and a profound lack of personal confidence in breastfeeding. When conceptualising their bodies in this way, as machines, the task was inevitably seen as demanding. The demanding nature of breastfeeding also related to the unpredictable way in which women's babies 'demanded' breast milk and thereby breached their once ordered temporal boundaries. In addition, the baby made indentations into their spatial and bodily boundaries. This disruption of boundaries resonates with the findings of Schmied and Barclay (1999). Women often felt wary of their baby 'depending' upon them in this way.

Women spoke repeatedly about breastfeeding as if it were simply breast milk feeding, a task that involved giving out and, as such, was experienced as demanding. Without the two-way reciprocity of a relationship, the act of providing for another could be experienced as depleting. Women placed a range of controls upon breastfeeding to support them in coping with their lack of confidence, fear of chaos and desire to plan for the future and return to 'normality'. Women were not only 'productive' but they also felt 'subjected' (Foucault 1977: 26) to temporal pressures and feelings of being under surveillance. Surveillance was experienced in relation to authoritative versions of 'correct breastfeeding'. Women also felt that they were under the 'gaze' because they were carrying out an intensely personal and culturally private activity in a highly public place. The hospital setting therefore magnified one of the major dilemmas for women in breastfeeding: the breaching of public–private boundaries. Women were very aware of their breastfeeding act as transgressing cultural norms that breasts were primarily sexual items.

Women expressed feelings of discord related to a 'natural' process often being experienced as emotionally and physically challenging. In the hospital setting, women were largely separated from family, friends and community networks at a time during which they were recovering from pregnancy and birth and coping with the newness of mothering a baby. They had to rapidly adapt to another place – the postnatal ward. Given this set of challenges they sought emotional support, encouragement and confidence-building. The encounters with midwives, in most cases, did very little to meet these needs and indeed were often counterproductive.

The midwives themselves felt 'productive' yet 'subjected'. They were heavily constrained by linear time, in that their work was unpredictable and rushed, coping with women who were usually complete or almost complete strangers. Their work was like that of production line workers: time pressured, routine, disconnected, fragmented and unsatisfying. In this context they saw themselves as 'supplying' a service under extremely 'demanding' conditions. Despite the pressures, they persevered day after day. Like the breastfeeding women, their work was conducted 'out of relationship' or relational context and this meant that their actions were seen as 'one-way' and therefore draining. Midwives engaged in ways of coping with the pressure and chaos. This included adopting rituals and routines and approaching women in disconnected, monologic, directive and managerial ways. The focus appeared to be upon the needs of the institution first, women and babies second.

The parallels between women 'supplying' breast milk and midwives 'supplying' a service are immediately both striking and alarming. The inevitable consequences for the postnatal women were that their needs for support were largely unmet. Equally, midwives' needs were met neither through the organisations nor through their relationships.

## Rethinking breastfeeding bodies

Breastfeeding is undoubtedly an embodied experience and in discussing women's bodies I am ever mindful of the well-rehearsed but little resolved dualistic feminist debates related to sameness or difference. These debates focus upon women's dilemmas as to whether they would prefer to strive to be recognised and respected for their differences or sameness in relation to men (Humm 1992; Van Esterik 1994; Shildrick 1997). As Shildrick (1997) argues, whichever of the positions are held, women may be blamed for their inadequacies as individuals and seen as inferior to men and the 'male prototype' (31), and 'whatever forms the dominant representation has taken, the bodies of women, whether all too present or disconcertingly absent, have served to ground the devaluation of women by men' (14). Shildrick (1997) proposes that it is the 'body itself, in whatever physical form it is experienced, that positions women as both morally deficient and existentially disabled' (14).

As I have discussed, breastfeeding creates particular dilemmas for feminists with regards to the sameness or difference debate (Van Esterik 1994; Carter 1995; Schmied 1998; Galtry 1997a, 1997b, 1997c, 2000; Blum 1999). Breastfeeding is a culturally mediated bio-psychosocial activity and, as such, there is an interaction between the physical body and social world. I have highlighted the ways in which women's bodily experiences appear to be heavily influenced by the concept of public place production, both conceptually and in the sense that the imperative to 'work', at least partially, influenced their plans during the first days of breastfeeding. Women often saw their bodies as being a means of production and yet they seemed to be strangely alienated from the product, describing to me a striking lack of trust or confidence in their body's ability to 'produce' milk. The demanding nature of breastfeeding and the imperative to plan for the future contributed to this distancing.

I therefore contend that women's experiences represent an extension of Martin's (1987) industrial model applied to labouring women. Like the labouring women, the breastfeeding women expressed alienation and separation from the production process (breastfeeding) and from the product of their labour (breast milk). While the breasts replaced the uterus as the operational machines, women profoundly doubted their ability to produce and deliver the product effectively, efficiently, on time and in the right measures. Given the limitations of women's 'machinery', management and control was required and this was conducted by the hospital midwives, referred to by Kirkham (1989) in her labour ward study as 'shop floor workers' (132). The baby, conceptualised as the consumer, was also seen as separate and indeed independent. The alienation and separation from both women's bodies and their babies was reinforced by being in a highly public, unfamiliar place, surrounded by unknown people. Women are clearly engaged in a 'productive' project and I suggest that part of this involves creating a dependent consumer paradoxically capable of early independence from her/his mother. Bottle feeding with formula milk marks progress in this direction. In this way women engage in the construction of citizens that will be relatively comfortable with the corporate control over food production, supply, purchasing and consumption, in line with capitalist ideology.

Having extended Martin's (1987) model from a labour situation to a breastfeeding situation, I further elaborate upon the model in several ways. While Martin (1987) referred to women's bodies being monitored by machinery, she did not extend this to incorporate Foucault's (1977) perspective on surveillance. She does refer to Foucault's (1977) discussion regarding *dismemberment* of the body, asserting that it has not slackened, but simply 'moved from the law to science' (21). I add complexity to the notion of productive bodies by introducing the concomitant concept of the 'subjected' body (Foucault 1977). Second, I focus in parallel on the productive experiences of the 'shop-floor workers' and highlight the ways that the culture within which midwives work contributes to both their own and the postnatal women's disconnected and alienating experiences.

I see the combination of doubt and mistrust in women's bodies and the concomitant use of those same bodies in the public domain – fuelling the capitalist economy, often under exploitative conditions as intricately connected with patriarchal dominance. I am passionate about seeing an increase in trust in women's bodies by women themselves and others in relation to breastfeeding. Women could then come to recognise and celebrate the concepts of embodiment, relationality and caring/nurturance. As Blum (1999) argues, this requires a collective effort by women to erode the dominant, male-orientated base metaphors applied to our bodies away from those centring on efficient production. However, as part of a collective project of re-establishing trust in ourselves as women, our bodies and the art of breastfeeding, we need to avoid returning to a form of essentialism that simply binds women to reproduction. This requires theorising new forms of female embodiment, as argued by Shildrick (1997):

> The move towards embodied selves need not entail a new form of essentialism nor a covert recuperation of biological determinism. Rather it celebrates embodiment as process, and speaks both to the refusal to split body and mind, and to the refusal to allow ourselves to be either normalised or pathologised. At the same time to stress both particularity and substantiality for the female body challenges the universalised male standard and opens up for us new possibilities of (well) being-in-the-world.
>
> (Shildrick 1997: 61)

If women's bodies are inscribed, at least in part, by powerful notions of efficient production and linear time then a crucial aspect of rethinking 'breastfeeding bodies' stems from a re-conceptualisation of time, to which I now turn.

## Re-conceptualising time

Women's experiences of breastfeeding were heavily influenced by linear time and the associated pressures. Women were coping at the same time with the past, present and future. They were coping with the past events of pregnancy, and previous experiences of mothering in some cases, and their more immediate experience of labour and birth. They were living in the present with all of the pressing matters of new motherhood and breastfeeding. Most striking was the way in which women expressed the linear sense of time running on and out. Breastfeeding was then experienced as time-consuming, and impeding, or potentially impeding, more pressing calls upon their time. The sense of urgency in relation to time was powerfully reinforced by the ways in which midwives communicated their own time pressures to women. This required women to compete for time in order to protect themselves from time 'going' elsewhere.

The conceptual lens through which I viewed women's accounts stemmed from the contrasting notions of cyclical and linear time (Cipolla 1967; Kahn 1989; Adam 1992; Bellaby 1992; Helman 1992; Starkey 1992). As Kahn (1989) asserts, linear time is so deeply embedded within western culture that any other notion of time is rarely considered. It is a time that is pitched relentlessly towards the future and is centred upon the notion of efficient production. Cyclical time, Kahn (1989) argues, is a bodily, rhythmic time that is a part of one's ontology and not separate and 'outside' like linear time. Whilst I agree with Kahn's differentiation between linear and cyclical time, I suggest that linear time has indeed become a powerful part of women's being or ontology. This requires me to shift in the direction of Foucault's (1977) theorising on time, in that he states 'time penetrates the body and with it all the meticulous controls of power' (152).

However, unlike Foucault, I argue that we *can* re-conceptualise time and in turn change our ontology. After all, if some of the limits or constraints upon women's time were lifted ... for a time ... then their perceptions of their breastfeeding bodies would, I believe, also change. Breastfeeding would not be seen as simply using up time and taking time from other activities. Kahn's (1989) notion of maialogical time, I believe, has enormous possibilities for changing our understanding of time and for restoring time for women to engage in breastfeeding their baby in a more fulfilling way. However, as she again asserts, maialogical time may be seen as part of 'birth time' for women but it may not be helpful for them to feel that it must continue throughout motherhood. This could recreate the tensions around essentialist notions of mothers being confined to the childcare role, the so-called 'full time earth mother' (31). She argues that:

> Uncorseting our maternal bodies does not have to be incompatible with living in linear time, providing that this time moves forward more slowly and with more digressions. Thus there would be time out for children [...]. Perhaps the time will come when both productive and reproductive labour will be honoured equally. Not the tokenism of Mother's Day, but an appreciation expressed through the reorganisation of work structures to accommodate the uncorseted maternal body.
>
> (Kahn 1989: 31)

Forman (1989) likewise argues that feminisation of women's time should 'resist the definition of woman as nature'. It should not mean a return to a form of 'lunar consciousness nor a celebration of women's natural cycle' (7, 8). Simonds (2002) also argues for changing conceptualisations of time as she warns us against the strictures imposed by the medical model's clock:

> Time is not only money, as the well-known aphorism claims. It is also power. If we take the time to reconsider these models, perhaps with time, demystification may lead us toward the re-conceptualisation of procreative time and the enhancement of procreative experiences.
>
> (Simonds 2002: 569)

Political activity is needed to restore the possibilities for women to take 'time-out' for mothering and breastfeeding, should they wish to do this. This requires a concerted effort with regard to national policies, as the global pattern of increasing numbers of mothers returning to paid employment creates dilemmas for women as they juggle the demands upon their time and bodies (Blum 1999; Galtry 2003). As Galtry (2003) cogently argues, extensive, well-paid, flexible and inclusive maternity leave provision combined with child-friendly workplace practices reduces tensions and dilemmas for women between reproductive and industrially productive activities.

The Scandinavian countries have led the way amongst industrialised countries in improving maternity rights, pay and workplace flexibility through statutory processes. These policies have had a marked impact upon the duration for which women breastfeed within Scandinavian countries (Austveg and Sundby 1995; Gerrard 2001; Galtry 2003). Clearly such statutory recognition sends powerful messages related to valuing parenting. Recent extensions to UK maternity pay and leave, in line with European Community guidelines, reflect a positive move that reduces penalties upon vulnerable low-paid part-time workers, whose rights were often very limited. Prior to these changes, a third of women returned to work before the end of their eighteen weeks of statutory maternity leave end because they couldn't afford to stay off work (Maternity Alliance 2003).

However, providing women with 'more time' will not necessarily lead to an automatic re-conceptualisation of time. This would require, as Adam (1992) states, recognition of the:

> Difference and the continuity between the times of becoming and the time of created invariability, the times of life and the times of death. We need to lift time from the level of the taken-for-granted meaning to an understanding that knows the relation between the finite resource, birth–death and being–becoming, between chronology, the seasons and growth. We need to de-alienate time: reconnect clock time to its sources and recognise its created machine character.
>
> (Adam 1992: 163)

With this recognition, women, as Forman and Sowton (1989) argue, could be encouraged to seek to subvert the power of time over their bodies by creating rhythms of their own. Merleau-Ponty (1962) likewise argues that time needs to be understood as a dimension of our being and not as a transfer upon ourselves of a phenomenon that is external. It would be tempting to suggest that midwives could assist women in re-conceptualising time in this way, so that there is an opening up of possibilities for women as they embark on motherhood. However, midwives would need to reflect on the ways in which *they* are controlled by time and indeed control time to even begin to engage with women on this issue. Sadly, for midwives on a busy maternity ward, there are powerful constraints of linear time upon their own bodies as they work in settings that resemble early factories. They are subjected not only to pressing linear time, but also to an experience of unpredictability, so that they never know at any time how much or how little time they may have to complete their tasks.

It needs to be remembered that, as Lynch (2002) argues, 'hospitals are organised as corporate work places overseen by managers whose job is to economise health care and in the case of privatised health care, make a profit' (180). Within this model, as demand outstrips supply, like other public services, hospitals are always likely to be under-resourced and it is the personal aspect of the service that is usually sacrificed. As Lipsky (1980) states, 'there are several ways in which street level bureaucracies characteristically provide fewer resources than necessary for workers to do their jobs adequately. The two most important are the ratio of workers to clients or cases and time' (29).

Unrelenting pressure upon midwives' time is a key source of oppression. As Lynch (2002) argues, we have lost our understanding of the 'rhythm of work and rest', of 'being' as well as 'doing', of recognising the need for 'spaces of contemplation, meditation and mediation' (184). The political ramifications of the pressures upon midwives' time are enormous and pressing. The growing literature that relates to the misery experienced by many midwives working within UK maternity hospitals illustrates this only too vividly (Kirkham 1999; Woodward 2000; Kirkham and Stapleton 2001b; Ball *et al.* 2002; Hughes *et al.* 2002; Deery 2003). Midwives are currently the main group of health workers and supporters of women during the postnatal period. Therefore, urgent political action is required to radically restructure the current maternity 'system' in the UK to address the now clear understanding that midwives as an oppressed and disempowered group are in turn disempowering women.

A re-conceptualisation of women's time – of both midwives and mothers – would be an essential part of any transformative action. There would need to be recognition that women need time in order to give time to others. This, in turn, requires recognition that caring time is cyclical and rhythmical allowing for relationality, sociability, mutuality and reciprocity. A crucial aspect of reorganising the maternity system would necessarily require a re-visioning of midwife–mother relationships and I believe that in turn this would support a re-visioning of early mother–baby relationships, issues I now turn to.

## Re-visioning relationships

Human experience in any situation is hugely impacted upon by relationships (Merleau-Ponty 1962) and these appear to be particularly influential during periods of emotional vulnerability, with new motherhood being a striking example (Ball 1994; Halldorsdottir and Karlsdottir 1996b; Barclay *et al.* 1997; Fenwick *et al.* 2000, 2001). Through observing and listening to women and midwives in an institutionalised maternity setting, I have been able to add to the existing body of knowledge centring upon the nature of encounters between midwives and service users (Kirkham 1989, 1993, 1997a; Halldorsdottir and Karlsdottir 1996b; Fenwick *et al.* 1999, 2000, 2001; Lock 1999; Lock and Gibb 2003).

The majority of encounters I observed resonated strongly with inhibitive nursing actions, referred to by Fenwick *et al.* (2000, 2001). However, I further elaborate upon the nature of 'caring/uncaring' encounters by critically highlighting the nature of the culture within which midwives were working, thus connecting with and extending the focus of other critical accounts within midwifery (Kirkham 1999; Woodward 2000; Kirkham and Stapleton 2001b; Ball *et al.* 2002; Hughes *et al.* 2002). The ritualistic, routinised, disconnected and managerial approaches of most midwives reflected, at least in part, their inability to gain any satisfaction through relationships with women. The tyranny of being under constant pressure of linear time combined with intense unpredictability was an additional but central component to midwives' emotion work. Midwives developed satisfaction through completing tasks, getting through the work and indeed getting off duty. Taking this analysis further I focus upon the striking parallels between breastfeeding women and midwives, with regard to the constraints upon them, in experiencing relationality within the maternity ward context.

The women were subjected to superficial, formal, intermittent and time-pressured encounters at a time when they were very emotionally vulnerable and lacking in confidence with breastfeeding. Through highlighting encounters that create situations in which women feel emotionally supported, encouraged and validated, I have identified interactions that went some way in supporting women in meeting the challenges they faced when breastfeeding during the early days. However, as I have highlighted, the individuals who engaged in this form of encounter struggled to create a relational context within which to achieve this. This was highly challenging within a cultural milieu in which midwives were primarily attending to the requirements of the institution rather than those of the women (Lock 1999; Kirkham and Stapleton 2001b; Shallow 2001a, 2001b, 2001c, 2001d; Ball *et al.* 2002; Hunter 2002, 2004; Deery 2003; Lock and Gibb 2003).

The breastfeeding woman enters another new form of relationality, with her baby, that of intimately sharing her body with another (Hewat and Ellis 1984; Bottorff 1990; Wrigley and Hutchinson 1990; Driscoll 1992; Leff *et al.* 1994; Dignam 1994; Lock 1999; Schmeid and Barclay 1999; Shaw 2003). This relationship may be experienced by women as a harmony, synchrony and mutuality (Hewat and Ellis 1984; Bottorff 1990; Wrigley and Hutchinson 1990; Leff *et al.* 1994; Schmeid and Barclay 1999). However, from my observations and through listening to women, I became aware that women's relationships with their babies were commonly placed 'on hold' while on the maternity wards. There was a striking absence of a sense of breastfeeding as a relationship between mother and baby. Relationship was rarely spoken about between mother and midwife or to me during conversations and interviews. This silence on relationships related in part to the way in which women conceptualised their bodies and breastfeeding, as discussed.

Breastfeeding a baby in a public place, surrounded by strangers and having to constantly compete for a midwife's time and attention, created counterproductive conditions to the building of women's confidence and to their sense of emotional well-being, both important to the development of a relationship with one's baby. The absence of reinforcing and validating midwife–mother relationships while in hospital appeared to contribute to a delay in early mother–child interaction, as referred to by others (Lock 1999; Fenwick *et al.* 2000, 2001). As I have stated, if midwives are unable to relate to women in a relational context they are unlikely to inculcate a positive relational feeling in women.

The parallels and connections between midwives and breastfeeding women are immediately striking in that any sense of 'giving' both by mothers (to their babies) and by midwives (to women) in the maternity ward setting was experienced as largely one-way and therefore draining. So how may we move away from this situation? If midwives were able to experience relationality with women they would not only 'give' but also receive emotionally (Hunter 2002, 2004). Likewise, if women could go beyond the one-way notion of 'giving out' to their baby and conceptualise breastfeeding in a more symmetrical relational context, then giving to a baby would be seen as part of a reciprocal relationship in which the mother also receives. This would both require and support a move away from women simply seeing themselves as labourers whose machines (breasts) may be emptied and refilled in order to supply the consumer.

As argued by others (Carter 1995; Schmied 1998; Blum 1999), I do not wish to create an essentialist meta-narrative that implies that all women should experience breastfeeding in positive relational terms during the early days of breastfeeding. However, I believe that within a supportive culture to include caring relationships, women would be more likely to experience relationality with their babies. I argue that for this to be actualised while in hospital, then a meaningful relationship between mother and midwife must be made possible. Given the time constraints upon midwives within the maternity ward settings, it may be appropriate to mobilise alternative forms of support for women while in hospital, as an interim solution. This may include employing mother-to-mother breastfeeding supporters to provide additional and focused support to breastfeeding women while on maternity wards. Peer supporter involvement on postnatal wards holds promise in that it restores a sense of community network support to an institutionalised setting, as described by Merewood and Philipp (2003).

Moving to a more radical position, from my analysis and that of others in related contexts (Lipsky 1980; Hunter 2002, 2004), it seems unlikely that 'tinkering' with the current system of institutionalised postnatal care will achieve much in changing the situation for women. The maternity ward culture, as described, is prohibitive to the shift to a relational conceptualisation. I therefore argue for a radical reappraisal of midwifery practice to enable the forming of meaningful relationships between mothers and midwives at this emotionally vulnerable time for women.

It seems that midwives exert peer pressure upon each other in an attempt to maintain institutional status quo (Kirkham 1999; Ball *et al.* 2002; Hunter 2002, 2004 Deery 2003). Therefore, to change a culture it seems unlikely that encouraging individuals to change their practice will be successful. We need collective resistance and transformational change to introduce models of postnatal care that enable midwives to engage with women meaningfully, in relationship and with sufficient time to do so. This can only be achieved via strong and collective actions through midwifery networks and organisations. Reflective practice groups, otherwise referred to as clinical supervision networks, would appear to be a clear way forward, as advocated by others (Deery 1999, 2003; Woodward 2000; Clarke and Wilcockson 2001, 2002; Hunter 2002, 2004). These groups offer a mechanism within practice settings whereby teams of midwives or nurses are facilitated in discussing models of care, reflections upon practice and issues of concern. The term 'clinical supervision' is rather unfortunate in its connections with notions of surveillance. I therefore prefer the label reflective practice group.

I now proceed to argue that the ways in which breastfeeding knowledge is generated and 'delivered' require reconfiguration.

## Reconfiguring knowledge

In Chapters 1 and 2, I highlighted the impact of Enlightenment thought, with its rationalistic and dualistic underpinnings upon the development of knowledge regarding the body and women's (re)productive and infant feeding practices. I argued that the techno-medical model reached an authoritative status that systematically and progressively subordinated other knowledges, in particular those held through the traditional, collective and embodied experiences of women within specific cultures and communities. The powerful 'authenticity' of the scientifically based knowledge supported the construction of a professional expertise and prowess that became increasingly difficult to challenge. As Jordan (1997) states, 'the power of authoritative knowledge is not that it is correct but that it counts' (58). However, as I have illustrated, over the past century there have been major fluctuations in what is considered to be 'authoritative' knowledge regarding infant feeding. This is exemplified in the current juxtaposition of baby-led/demand feeding advocates with those who continue to recommend the imposition of control and routines for babies.

The most striking oscillation in authoritative knowledges may be seen in the attempts this decade to reverse the medically advocated regimentation of breastfeeding based on new understandings of the physiology of breastfeeding. There is a huge and growing body of research highlighting that breastfeeding confers physiological benefits upon the mother and child (Wilson *et al.* 1998; Anderson *et al.* 1999; Oddy *et al.* 1999). There is also a growing understanding of the ways in which breastfeeding women may be supported in effectively attaching their baby to their breast in a way that enhances the physiological process of lactation, satiates the baby and minimises nipple trauma (Woolridge 1986a, 1986b, 1995; Righard and Alade 1992; Renfrew *et al.* 2000). This issue, as stated, is often bypassed within sociological critiques and yet it is embraced by the voluntary breastfeeding organisations, in that they pay considerable attention to supporting women with attachment and effective feeding practices. Indeed, it seems that women are highly appreciative of skilled support with breastfeeding from mother-to-mother breastfeeding supporters (Dykes 2003). However, a fundamental difference lies in the approaches adopted by voluntary supporters. They adopt a person-centred, dialogic and individualised approach that acknowledges the importance of women's experiential and embodied knowledge. This means that they engage with women's agendas and tailor the principles of effective breastfeeding to women's individual needs.

By contrast, when breastfeeding information and support is provided in hospital, by midwives, it is commonly issued in a routinised, prescriptive, authoritative manner that disregards the personal agenda of the woman. The encounters tend to be time-pressured and monologic. This approach conforms to the techno-medical ideology which, as Doyal and Pennell (1981) state, emphasises 'the physical and the quantifiable at the expense of the psychological and phenomenological' (226). The resulting inequality in power renders two-way dialogue between equals almost impossible to fulfil (Kirkham 1993; Stapleton *et al.* 2002b). The professional is assumed to have the expert and authoritative knowledge and the mother to be a passive recipient of the wisdom imparted (Jordan 1997; Edwards 2000, 2005). This authoritative approach within a setting in which women have to compete for midwives' limited time contributes to their emotional vulnerability. The didactic approach of the midwives also contributes towards an undermining of women's confidence in their bodies and their ability to breastfeed. Of even more concern is the situation that Cronk (2000) describes whereby the 'power over women' which accompanies this transmission of authoritative knowledge at the beginning of their experience of parenting may contribute to an ongoing process of female disempowerment (23).

There is now a major emphasis upon the promotion of breastfeeding as a public health issue with the provision of information on the health benefits of breastfeeding being central. While there is indeed a substantial basis for the provision of this information it is often not counterbalanced by effective support for women. Therefore, women appear to be commencing breastfeeding in hospital, influenced by the strong promotional messages, but are then conducting breastfeeding within an environment that resembles a factory production line with little in the way of a supportive infrastructure. This imbalance between promotion and effective support appears to be problematic for women's emotional well-being and sense of personal confidence with breastfeeding.

Knowledge about breastfeeding generated through scientific methods should not be disregarded simply because it stems from techno-medical disciplines. However, such knowledge should not be considered as more legitimate than women's embodied knowledge simply because it constitutes 'evidence-based' enquiry. Insights from this field have a place, but their position must be alongside, and not above, the knowledges generated through the experiences and accounts of women. The meanings of breastfeeding for women may be presented as they stand without theorising (Brown and McPherson 1998) or within theoretical frameworks. These knowledges need to take account of the embodied, emotional and social nature of breastfeeding, the ways in which women negotiate breastfeeding in a range of cultural contexts, and the macro-political influences upon women in relation to their infant feeding patterns.

Midwives involved in supporting breastfeeding women have much to learn from women's experiential and embodied knowledges and from the voluntary breastfeeding support organisations. This requires that midwives are facilitated in exploring their own personal and vicarious experiences of breastfeeding, as argued by Battersby (1999, 2002), so that they may use 'self' when appropriate and in ways that support rather than undermine. Midwives would then be more likely to respect knowledge generated from women's personal and embodied experiences. Midwives would require a working knowledge of person-centred counselling to include learning to listen to women and a concomitant knowledge of the principles underpinning effective breastfeeding. By combining person-centred counselling with supporting effective breastfeeding, women's individual needs may be met while at the same time information that is supportive to them is provided effectively and in dialogue. In this way, the principles of effective breastfeeding constitute a guide not a prescription and support confidence-building and encouragement.

There needs to be implementation of mechanisms to support midwives in reflective practice that enables them to collectively consider the issues related to supporting breastfeeding women and the implications of their practice. This need to address the reflexive cycle of professional practice, as recommended by others, could take place via reflective practice groups and within midwifery education (Deery 1999, 2003; Woodward 2000; Battersby 2002; Clarke and Wilcockson 2001, 2002; Hunter 2002, 2004). The approach to this should facilitate not simply personal reflection upon practice but also critical engagement with broader socio-political issues (Hunter 2002, 2004), thus allowing for collective understandings of limit situations and limit acts (Freire 1972).

However, having observed the settings within which midwives are charged with the role of supporting women, I argue that it is pointless to simply target midwives with these messages. While the educational programmes and clinical supervision networks should be utilised to facilitate midwives in developing the skills to support women in effective ways, this is still only a part of the picture. To educate midwives in this way and then release them into current hospital-based environments, like the ones I describe, may simply raise their levels of dissonance and dissatisfaction. I therefore now argue for a more radical agenda that offers real alternatives to midwives and women through the provision of non-institutionalised postnatal settings.

## Relocating place and space

The emphasis upon spatiality as part of human experience (Merleau-Ponty 1962; Berger and Luckmann 1966) has gained growing attention as medical geographers (Pain *et al.* 2001; Cartier 2002; Mahon-Daly and Andrews 2002); sociologists (Casey 2003; Halford and Leonard 2003) and midwives (Schmied 1998; Schmied and Barclay 1999; Lock and Gibb 2003) focus attention upon space and place in the health service.

This ethnographic account illustrates the ways in which women's spatial boundaries were dramatically redefined as they shared their external body and internal fluids with their baby through breastfeeding. This contributed to women's perceptions that their baby was demanding, given their conceptualisation of breastfeeding as a transfer of nutrients. Additional time at the breast was seen as the baby using the woman as a 'dummy'. Women endeavoured to retain some personal identity and space, within a public place, with the curtains utilised as a barrier. However, in reality they had little claim to any space and were subjected to strangers entering their personal space in unpredictable ways to include moving into their bodily space through handling of their breasts and related activities associated with postnatal care. In addition, women were obliged to breastfeed in a public place, contributing to feelings of dissonance and requiring considerable personal negotiation of their space. Both mothers and midwives came under a powerful gaze in this public setting (Foucault 1980).

The hospital is not the mother's territory and therefore can never become like home, despite attention to architecture and furnishings. It is a place where women are removed from their community, where medical management is super-valued and rituals and routines thrive. The institutional orientation created by hospital settings inevitably reduces relationality and woman-centredness, as demonstrated by others (Lock 1999; Allan 2001; Kirkham and Stapleton 2001b; Shallow 2001a, 2001b, 2001c, 2001d; Ball et al. 2002; Hunter 2002, 2004; Deery 2003; Lock and Gibb 2003). Lock and Gibb (2003) highlight the enormous power of the hospital place over both midwives and women. As they assert, it a place of physical, emotional and spiritual alienation and is therefore counterproductive to independence, confidence and emotional recuperation for women. While hospital may be seen as a place of safety, should something 'go wrong', as Lock (1999) argues, it is not emotionally safe.

In focusing upon women's embodied experiences, the power of linear time, authoritative knowledges and relationships, I challenge the suitability of the hospital, as described here, as the place in which women begin to establish breastfeeding. I also challenge the suitability of hospital as a place for birthing for the majority of women and, if this issue were to be addressed, women would receive their entire postnatal care in the home following birthing either in their own home or in a birth centre. I also advocate independent midwifery as an alternative to the current system, in that even when working in the community midwives are still somewhat accountable to their nearby institution, as cogently illustrated by Edwards (2000, 2001, 2005). However, the discussion here relates to women who continue to birth in hospital. I believe that it is now time to radically change the place in which postnatal support for women is provided. While a hospital setting will always be required for some women and desired by others, if an appealing alternative was offered then women might well opt for it. I argue that women could be offered postnatal care in their own home, but with increased support. The savings in resources by de-medicalising postnatal care would enable a relocation of resources to community care.

Studies have failed to show any advantage with regard to breastfeeding duration when comparing standard hospital postnatal care to early discharge and care in the community (Waldenstrom et al. 1987; Svedulf 1998; Margolis and Schwartz 2000; Winterburn and Fraser 2000; Sheehan et al. 2001; McKeever et al. 2002; Brown et al. 2003). However, it is clear within these studies that women appreciated the one-to-one support with breastfeeding provided in their own home in addition to the aspects of comfort, privacy and rejoining their family. While these studies all employed a nurse or midwife to provide the additional community support, this is not the only model available. Breastfeeding peer support schemes are becoming increasingly recognised as an effective way to protect, promote and support the practice of breastfeeding in communities around the world (Dykes 2003, 2005a; Sikorski *et al.* 2004; WHO 2003).

## For such a time as this ...

Women's breastfeeding experiences are influenced by their corporeality, temporality, breastfeeding knowledge(s), relationships and place. Within the hospital culture both breastfeeding women and midwives are engaged in 'productive' activities under considerable emotional pressure in a highly public place, open to many observers. Women experience dissonance as reality and expectation clash and they accommodate and/or resist authoritative knowledges, cultural ambiguities and associated surveillance of their bodies within public places. The hospital constitutes a place in which linear time is always in 'short supply', yet reified and randomised, creating challenges for mothers and midwives in coping with their daily activities. 'Supplying' for another's needs within a cultural milieu, and indeed macro-culture, in which linear temporal pressures are magnified and possibilities for relationality minimised, leads to both breastfeeding women and midwives experiencing their work as 'demanding'. While being demanded upon remains the predominant feeling, breastfeeding will continue to be seen as short term, marginal and disruptive, as will the act of 'caring' by midwives. Both then have to construct ways of coping with and controlling their situation. The nature of the encounters between mothers and midwives within hospital reflects the time-driven, rule-bound, institutional orientation of midwives and the ways in which both groups feel the pressure and cope with chaos. Both breastfeeding women and midwives are indeed 'productive' yet 'subjected' in this setting.

I seek to represent the experiences of breastfeeding women as an integrated paradigm in several ways. First, the hospital-based study reflects the complexity of women's experiences of breastfeeding and their active participation in negotiating this experience within a specific cultural milieu. This micro-perspective that stems from the meanings for women when engaging in a breastfeeding 'project' in hospital settings is then contextualised within a macro-political economic perspective. The latter highlights the constraints upon breastfeeding women in relation to continued medical centralisation and management of (re)productive activities, the power of commercial influences, the reification of linear time and the devaluing of women's embodied experiences and relationality within a western patriarchal society. By combining the micro-perspective with the macro-perspective, the balance between recognition of individual agency and structural impositions is achieved.

I argue against purely essentialist notions that all women will be empowered to breastfeed, simply through socio-political and health practice reform. While I argue that social policy should indeed recognise the competing demands upon women and their need for flexible options with regard to their various forms of work, I also assert that full consideration needs to be given to the contemporary cultural context within which women breastfeed. This requires recognition of the embodied, emotional and social nature of breastfeeding and the ways in which women negotiate the experience. Thus, social policy should enable but not coerce women to breastfeed and the ways in which breastfeeding is promoted should strongly move away from maternal duty and essentialist notions of mothering. I argue for a balanced approach to promoting and supporting breastfeeding to allow for a considerable increase in support relative to promotion. This requires a clear redefining of breastfeeding as both a relational and a socially valued activity while moving away from a model in which the body becomes little more than a potentially dysfunctional machine producing, supplying and transferring nutrients to a consumer.

In combining theory with praxis, several issues need to be addressed – from social policy level through to breastfeeding supporter practices. Maternity legislation needs to enable women to have the time and space to engage in breastfeeding as an embodied activity, while still maintaining a career should they decide to. If women anticipated this 'time out' without financial loss then their postnatal period might be considerably less pressured. If women understood the concept of maialogical time and were able to incorporate it, at least partially, into their lives, they might feel less pressured about their babies' need to take their time. Perhaps it is time to rethink what constitutes liberation for women, and having time to work flexibly and experience relationality would be fundamental in any such review.

The ways in which breastfeeding knowledge is generated and circulated needs radical reappraisal. Evidence-based knowledge needs to be juxtaposed with community-based collective, embodied knowledge generated by women. A proliferation of community projects such as peer support schemes appears to offer a strong way forward in this community capacity-building endeavour (Fairbank et al. 2000; Dykes 2003, 2005c; Sikorski et al. 2004). Such schemes could constitute part of a relocation of women's postnatal care into the community.

It is inappropriate to simply make recommendations for midwives to implement, given that their practices are heavily constrained by social structures that impinge upon their corporeality, temporality, knowledge(s), relationships and physical spaces. Rather, professional and voluntary organisations need to be accessed and mobilised to lobby, lead and act as catalysts in changing the ways and places in which midwives are enabled to support women. While this action will take time, I argue that now is the time for this agenda to proceed.

# Bibliography

Aamodt, A. (1991) 'Ethnography and epistemology: generating nursing knowledge'. In: J. Morse (ed.) *Qualitative Nursing Research a Contemporary Dialogue* (pp. 40–53). London: Sage.

Aasheim, V., Dalhaug, R.E. and Vik, B. (2000) 'Breast-feeding in Norway'. *MIDIRS Midwifery Digest* 10 (3): 372–374.

Adair, L., Popkin, B. and Guilkey, D. (1993) 'The duration of breast feeding: how is it affected by biological, socio-demographic, health sector and food industry factors?' *Demography* 30 (1): 63–80.

Adam, B. (1992) 'Time and health implicated: a conceptual critique'. In: R. Frankenberg (ed.) *Time, Health and Medicine* (pp. 153–164). London: Sage.

Allan, H. (2001) 'A "good" enough nurse: supporting patients in a fertility clinic'. *Nursing Inquiry* 8: 51–60.

Alldred, P. (1998) 'Ethnography and discourse analysis – dilemmas in representing the voices of children'. In: J. Ribbens and R. Edwards (eds) *Feminist Dilemmas in Qualitative Research* (pp. 147–170). London: Sage.

Altergott, M. (1991) 'Artificial infant feeding: women's loss, men's gain'. *Issues in Reproductive and Genetic Engineering* 4 (2): 129–141.

Anderson, J.W., Johnstone, B.M. and Remley, D.T. (1999) 'Breast-feeding and cognitive development: a meta-analysis'. *American Journal of Clinical Nutrition* 70 (4): 525–535.

Anderson, T. (2000) 'Feeling safe enough to let go: the relationship between a woman and her midwife during the second stage of labour'. In: M. Kirkham (ed.) *The Midwife–Mother Relationship* (pp. 92–119). London: Macmillan.

Anderson, T. and Podkolinski, J. (2000) 'Reflections on midwifery care and the postnatal period'. In: J. Alexander, C. Roth and V. Levy (eds) *Midwifery Practice Core Topics 3 (Postnatal)*. London: MacMillan.

Apple, R. (1987) *Mothers and Medicine – A Social History of Infant Feeding 1890–1950*. London: The University of Wisconsin Press.

Appleton, J.V. (1995) 'Analysing qualitative interview data: addressing issues of validity and reliability'. *Journal of Advanced Nursing* 22: 993–997.

Arney, W.R. (1982) *Power and the Profession of Obstetrics*. London: The University of Chicago Press.

Association for Breastfeeding Mothers (2003) *Association for Breastfeeding Mothers Home Page*. At: http://beehive.thisissouthwales.co.uk/default.asp?WCI=SiteHome&ID=5823 (accessed 26 Sept 2003).

Association of Social Anthropologists of the UK and the Commonwealth (ASA) (1999) *Ethical Guidelines for Good Research Practice*. At: www.asa.anthropology.ac.uk/ethics2.html (accessed 4 March 2005).

Attride-Stirling, J. (2001) 'Thematic networks: an analytical tool for qualitative research'. *Qualitative Research* 1 (3): 385–405.

Audit Commission (1997) *First Class Delivery: Improving Maternity Services in England and Wales*. London: Audit Commission.

Auerbach, K. (1995) 'Breastfeeding as the "default" infant feeding'. *Journal of Human Lactation* 11 (2): 81–82.

Austveg, B. and Sundby, J. (1995) *Empowerment of Women: The Case of Breastfeeding in Norway*. Norway: Ammehjelpen.

Baer, E. (1982) 'Babies means business'. *New Internationalist* April: 22–23.

Ball, J.A. (1994) *Reactions to Motherhood. The Role of Postnatal Care* (2nd edn). Cheshire: Books for Midwives Press.

Ball L., Curtis P. and Kirkham M. (2002) *Why Do Midwives Leave?* Royal College of Midwives, London.

Balsamo, F., De Mari, G., Maher, V. and Serini, R. (1992) 'Production and pleasure: research on breastfeeding in Turin' In: 0.V Maher (ed.) *The Anthropology of Breastfeeding, Natural Law or Social Construct* (pp. 59–90). Oxford: Berg.

Bandura, A. (1995) 'Exercise of personal and collective efficacy in changing societies'. In: A. Bandura (ed.) *Self-efficacy in Changing Societies* (pp. 1–45). Cambridge: Cambridge University Press.

Barclay, L., Everitt, L., Rogan, F., Schmied, V. and Wyllie, A. (1997) 'Becoming a mother – an analysis of women's experience of early motherhood'. *Journal of Advanced Nursing* 25: 719–728.

Baron, R.A. and Byrne, D. (1991) *Social Psychology: Understanding Human Interaction*. London: Allyn and Bacon.

Bartlett, A. (2000) 'Thinking through breasts'. *Feminist theory* 1 (2): 173–188.

Bartlett, A. (2002) 'Breastfeeding as headwork: corporeal feminism and meaning for breastfeeding'. *Women's Studies International Forum* 885 (1): 1–10.

Battersby, S. (1999) 'Midwives' experiences of breastfeeding: can the attitudes developed affect midwives support and promote breastfeeding?' *Triennial Congress of the International Confederation of Midwives, Midwifery and Safe Motherhood beyond the year 2000 Book of Proceedings*. Manila, Phillipines, 22–27 May: 52–57.

Battersby, S. (2000) 'Breastfeeding and bullying – who's putting the pressure on?' *Practising Midwife* 3 (8): 36–38.

Battersby, S. (2001a) Simply the Breast: Evaluation of a Peer Support Programme. At: http://sheffield.ac.uk/surestart/brstfrnt.html (accessed 11 April 2003).

Battersby, S. (2001b) 'The wordly wise project: a different approach to breastfeeding support'. *Practising Midwife* 4 (6): 30–31.

Battersby, S. (2002) 'Midwives' embodied knowledge of breastfeeding'. *MIDIRS Midwifery Digest* 12 (4): 523–526.

Baumslag, N. and Michels, D.L. (1995) *Milk, Money and Madness – The Culture and Politics of Breastfeeding*. London: Bergin & Garvey.

Beake, S. and McCourt, C. (2002) 'Evaluation of the use of health care assistants to support disadvantaged women breastfeeding in the community'. Summary – DH funded project. In: F. Dykes (2003) *Infant Feeding Initiative: A Report Evaluating the Breastfeeding Practice Projects 1999–2002*. London: Department of Health.

Beeken, S. and Waterston, T. (1992) 'Health service support of breastfeeding – are we practising what we preach?' *British Medical Journal* 305: 285–289.

Beekman, D. (1977) *The Mechanical Baby. A Popular History of the Theory and Practice of Child Raising.* London: Dobson Books.

Begley, C.M. (2001) '"Giving midwifery care": student midwives' views of their working role'. *Midwifery* 17: 24–34.

Belenky, M.F., Clinchy, B.M., Goldberger, N.R. and Tarule, J.M. (1986) *Women's Ways of Knowing: The Development of Self, Voice and Mind.* New York: Basic Books.

Bellaby, P. (1992) 'Broken rhythms and unmet deadlines: workers' and managers' time-perspectives'. In: R. Frankenberg (ed.) *Time, Health and Medicine* (pp. 108–122). London: Sage.

Bellamy, R. (1995) 'The social and political thought of Antonio Gramsci'. In: A. Giddens, B. Held, D. Hubert, D Seymour and J. Thompson (eds) *The Polity Reader of Social Theory* (pp. 32–37). Oxford: Polity Press.

Berg, M., Lundgren, I., Hermansson, E. and Wahlberg, V. (1996) 'Women's experience of the encounter with the midwife during childbirth'. *Midwifery* 12: 11–15.

Berger, P.L. and Luckmann, T. (1966) *The Social Construction of Reality: A Treatise in the Sociology of Knowledge.* Harmondsworth: Penguin.

Bergevin, Y., Dougherty, C. and Kramer, M. (1983) 'Do infant formula samples shorten the duration of breastfeeding?' *The Lancet,* 21 May: 1148–1151.

Bernaix, L.W. (2000) 'Nurses' attitudes, subjective norms, and behavioural intentions toward support of breastfeeding mothers'. *Journal of Human Lactation* 16 (3): 201–209.

Beynon, H. (1973) *Working for Ford.* Harmondsworth: Penguin.

Bibeau, G. (1988) 'A step toward thick thinking: from webs of significance to connections across dimensions'. *Medical Anthropology Quarterly* 2 (4): 402–416.

Blum, L.M. (1993) 'Mothers, babies and breastfeeding in late capitalist America: the shifting contexts of feminist theory'. *Feminist Studies* 19 (2): 291–311.

Blum, L.M. (1999) *At The Breast. Ideologies of Breastfeeding and Motherhood in the Contemporary United States.* Boston: Beacon Press.

Blyth, R., Creedy, D.K., Dennis, C-L., Moyle, W., Pratt, J. and De Vries (2002) 'Effect of maternal confidence on breastfeeding duration: an application of breastfeeding self-efficacy theory'. *BIRTH* 29 (4): 278–284.

Bobel, C.G. (2001) 'Bounded liberation – a focused study of La Leche League International'. *Gender & Society* 15 (1): 130–151.

Bondas-Salonen, T. (1998) 'New mothers' experiences of postpartum care – a phenomenological follow-up study'. *Journal of Clinical Nursing* 7 (2): 165–174.

Bottorff, J. (1990) 'Persistence in breastfeeding: a phenomenological investigation'. *Journal of Advanced Nursing* 15: 201–209.

Bowes, A. and Domokos, T.M. (1998) 'Negotiating breastfeeding: Pakistani women, white women and their experiences in hospital and at home'. *Sociological Research Online* 3 (3): 1–21. At: www.socresonline.org.uk/socresonline/3/3/5.html (accessed 24 March 04).

Bowling, A. (1997) *Research Methods in Health. Investigating Health and Health Services.* Buckingham: Open University Press.

Boyle, J. (1994) 'Styles of ethnography'. In: J. Morse (ed.) *Critical Issues in Qualitative Research Methods* (pp. 158–159). Thousand Oaks, California: Sage.

Bradley, J.E. and Meme, J. (1992) 'Breastfeeding promotion in Kenya: changes in health worker knowledge, attitude and practices 1982–1989'. *Journal of Tropical Pediatrics* 38: 228–234.

Bramwell, R. (2001) 'Blood and milk: constructions of female bodily fluids in western society'. *Women and Health* 34 (4): 85–96.

Breastfeeding Network (2003) *Who We Are: History*. At: http://www.breastfeeding network.org.uk/whoweare/history.html (accessed 26 Sept 2003).

Brink, P. and Edgecombe, N. (2003) 'What is becoming of ethnography?' *Qualitative Health Research* 13 (7): 1028–1030.

Briscoe, L., Lavender, T. and Alfirevic, Z. (2002) 'Supporting women after obstetric complications'. *British Journal of Midwifery* 10 (10): 620–625.

Britton, C. (1997) '"Letting it go, letting it flow": women's experiential accounts of the let-down reflex'. *Social Sciences in Health* 3 (3): 176–187.

Britton, C. (1998) 'The influence of antenatal information on breastfeeding experiences'. *British Journal of Midwifery* 6 (5): 312–315.

Brown, A.B. and McPherson, K.R. (eds) (1998) *The Reality of Breastfeeding Reflections by Contemporary Women*. London: Bergin and Garvey.

Brown, S., Small, R., Faber, B., Krastev, A. and Davis, P. (2003) 'Early postnatal discharge from hospital for healthy mothers and term infants' (Cochrane Review). In: *The Cochrane Library*, issue 4. Chichester: John Wiley & Sons.

Brunner, E. (1996) 'The social and biological basis of cardiovascular disease in office workers'. In: D. Blane, E. Brunner and R. Wilkinson (eds) *Health and Social Organisation, Towards a Health Policy for the 21st Century* (pp. 272–302). London: Routledge.

Budin, P. (1907) *The Nursling*. London: Caxton.

Burden, B. (1998) 'Privacy or help? The use of curtain positioning strategies within the maternity ward environment as a means of achieving and maintaining privacy, or as a form of signalling to peers and professionals in an attempt to seek information or support'. *Journal of Advanced Nursing* 27: 15–23.

Burman, E. (1992) 'Feminism and discourse in developmental psychology: power, subjectivity and interpretation'. *Feminism & Psychology* 2 (1): 45–60.

Carson, C. (2001) 'How is the government going to raise breast-feeding rates?' *British Journal of Midwifery* 9 (5): 292–293.

Carter, P. (1995) *Feminism, Breasts and Breastfeeding*, London: Macmillan.

Cartier, C. (2002) 'From home to hospital and back again: economic restructuring, end of life, and the gendered problems of place-switching health services'. *Social Science and Medicine* 56: 2289–2301.

Casey, E.S. (2003) 'From space to place in contemporary health care'. *Social Science and Medicine* 56: 2245–2247.

Cattaneo, A. and Buzzetti, R. (2001) 'Effect on rates of breast feeding of training for the Baby Friendly Hospital Initiative'. *British Medical Journal* 323: 1358–1362.

Chalmers, J. (1991) 'Variations in breast feeding advice, a telephone survey of community midwives and health visitors'. *Midwifery*, 7: 162–166.

Chen, C-H., Wang, S-Y. and Chang, M-Y. (2001) 'Women's perceptions of helpful and unhelpful nursing behaviours during labour: a study in Taiwan'. *BIRTH* 28 (3): 180–185.

Chesney, M. (2001) 'Dilemmas of self in the method'. *Qualitative Health Research* 11 (1) 127–135.

Cipolla, C.M. (1967) *Clocks and Culture 1300–1700*. London: Collins.

Clarke, C.L. and Wilcockson, J. (2001) 'Professional and organizational learning: analysing the relationship with the development of practice'. *Journal of Advanced Nursing* 34, 264–272.

Clarke, C.L. and Wilcockson, J. (2002) 'Seeing need and developing care: exploring knowledge for and from practice'. *International Journal of Nursing Studies* 39, 397–406.

Cloherty, M., Alexander, J., Holloway, I. and Galvin, K. (2004) *An Ethnography of the Supplementation of Breastfed Babies.* Bournemouth: Bournemouth University Press.

Colson, S. (1998a) 'Breastfeeding Nemesis'. *Midwifery Today* Winter 1998: 27–33.

Colson S. (1998b) 'Breastfeeding Editorial'. *Midwifery Today* Winter 1998: 34.

Colson, S.D., de Rooy, L. and Hawdon, J.M. (2003) 'Biological nurturing increases duration of breastfeeding for a vulnerable cohort'. *MIDIRS Midwifery Digest* 13 (1): 92–97.

Cooke, M., Sheehan, A. and Schmied, V. (2003) 'A description of the relationship between breastfeeding experiences, breastfeeding satisfaction, and weaning in the first 3 months after birth'. *Journal of Human Lactation* 19 (2): 145–156.

Corbin, J. and Strauss, A. (1990) 'Grounded theory research: procedures, canons and evaluative criteria'. *Qualitative Sociology* 13: 3–21.

Cox, S.G. and Turnbull, C.J. (1998) 'Developing effective interactions to improve breastfeeding outcomes'. *Breastfeeding Review* 6: 11–22.

Cregan, M.D. and Hartmann, P.E. (1999) 'Computerized breast measurement from conception to weaning: clinical implications'. *Journal of Human Lactation* 15 (2): 89–96.

Cronk, M. (2000) 'The Midwife: a professional servant?' In: M. Kirkham (ed.) *The Midwife-Mother Relationship* (pp. 19–27). London: Macmillan.

Crotty, M. (1998) *The Foundations of Social Research. Meaning and Perspective in the Research Process.* London: Sage.

Csordas, T. (1988) 'The conceptual status of hegemony and critique in medical anthropology'. *Medical Anthropology Quarterly* 2 (4): 416–421.

Csordas, T. (ed.) (1994a) *Embodiment and Experience: The Existential Ground of Culture and Self.* Cambridge: Cambridge University Press.

Csordas, T. (1994b) 'Introduction: the body as representation and being-in-the-world'. In: T. Csordas (ed.) *Embodiment and Experience: The Existential Ground of Culture and Self.* Cambridge: Cambridge University Press.

Cunningham, F.G., Grant, N.F., Leveno, K.J. and Gilstrap, L.C. (1993) Williams Obstetrics (19th edn). Stamford, CT: Appleton & Lange.

Curtis, P., Thomas, G., Stapleton, H. and Kirkham, S. (2001) 'Focus groups with childbearing women'. In: M. Kirkham and H. Stapleton (eds) *Informed Choice in Maternity Care: An Evaluation of Evidence Based Leaflets* (pp. 113–136). University of York: NHS Centre for Reviews and Dissemination.

Cuttini, M., Del Santo, M., Kaldor, K., Pavan, C., Rizzian, C. and Tonchella, C. (1995) 'Rooming-in, breastfeeding and mother's satisfaction in an Italian nursery'. *Journal of Reproductive & Infant Psychology* 13: 41–46.

Daly, J. and McDonald, I. (1992), 'Introduction: the problem as we saw it'. In: J. Daly, I. McDonald and E. Willis (eds) *Researching Health Care. Designs, Dilemmas, Disciplines.* London: Tavistock/Routledge.

Davies, R.M. and Atkinson, P. (1991) 'Students of midwifery: "doing the obs" and other coping strategies'. *Midwifery* 7: 113–121.

Davis-Floyd, R. (1992) *Birth as an American Rite of Passage.* London: University of California Press.

Davis-Floyd, R. (1994) 'The technocratic body: American childbirth as cultural expression'. *Social Science and Medicine* 38 (8): 1125–1140.

Davis-Floyd, R. (1998) 'From technobirth to cyborg babies – reflections on the emergent discourse of a holistic anthropologist'. In: R. Davis-Floyd and J. Dumit (eds) *Cyborg Babies: From Techno-Sex to Techno-Tots* (pp. 255–285). London: Routledge.

Davis-Floyd, R. and Dumit, J. (1998) *Cyborg Babies: From Techno-Sex to Techno-Tots*. London: Routledge.

Davis-Floyd, R. and Sargent, F. (eds) (1997*) Childbirth and Authoritative Knowledge: Cross-Cultural Perspectives*. London: University of California Press.

Davis-Floyd, R. and St John, G. (1998) *From Doctor to Healer: The Transformative Journey*. London: Rutgers University Press.

de Oliveira, M.I., Camacho, L.A.B. and Tedstone, A. (2001) 'Extending breastfeeding duration through primary care: a systematic review of prenatal and postnatal interventions'. *Journal of Human Lactation* 17 (4): 326–343.

Deery, R. (1999) 'Improving relationships through clinical supervision'. *British Journal of Midwifery* 7 (3): 160–163.

Deery, R. (2003) 'Engaging with clinical supervision in a community midwifery setting: an action research study'. Unpublished thesis, University of Sheffield.

Deery, R. (2005) 'An action-research study exploring midwives' support needs and the effect of group clinical supervision'. *Midwifery* 21: 161–176.

Denzin, N. and Lincoln, Y. (1994) 'Major paradigms and perspectives'. In: N. Denzin and Y. Lincoln (eds) *Handbook of Qualitative Research* (pp. 99–104). London: Sage.

Department of Health and Social Security (DHSS) (1974) *Present Day Practice in Infant Feeding*. Report of a Working Party of the Panel on Child Nutrition Committee on Medical Aspects of Food Policy. London: HMSO.

Department of Health and Social Security (DHSS) (1978) *Breastfeeding*. Committee on Medical Aspects of Food Policy: Panel on Child Nutrition. London: HMSO.

Department of Health and Social Security (DHSS) (1980) *Present Day Practice in Infant Feeding*. Report of a Working Party of the Panel on Child Nutrition Committee on Medical Aspects of Food Policy. London: HMSO.

Department of Health and Social Security (DHSS) (1988a) *Present Day Practice in Infant Feeding*. Third Report of a Working Party of the Panel on Child Nutrition Committee on Medical Aspects of Food Policy. London: HMSO.

Department of Health and Social Security (DHSS) (1988b) *Caring for the breastfeeding mother: the lost 25%*. Conference report. London: DHSS.

Department of Health (1993) *Changing Childbirth*. London: HMSO.

Department of Health (1994) *Weaning and the Weaning Diet*. Report of the working group of the Committee on Medical Aspects of Food Policy. London: HMSO.

Department of Health National Breastfeeding Working Group (1995) *Breastfeeding: Good Practice Guidance to the NHS*. London: Department of Health.

Department of Health (1999) *Saving Lives, Our Healthier Nation*. London: TSO.

Department of Health (2000) *The NHS Plan: Improving Health and Reducing Inequality*. London: Department of Health. At: http://www.nhs.uk/nationalplan/npch13.htm (accessed on 4 March 2003).

Department of Health (2002) *Improvement, Expansion and Reform: The Next Three Years' Priorities and Planning Framework, 2003–2006*. London: Department of Health. At: |FCO|Hyperlinkhttp://www.doh.gov.uk/planning2003–2006/index.htm |FCC|(accessed on 4 March 2003).

Department of Health (2005a) *Choosing Health: Making Healthy Choices Easier*. London: Department of Health.

Department of Health (2005b) *Choosing a Better Diet: A Food and Health Action Plan.* London: Department of Health.

Dettwyler, K. (1987). 'Breastfeeding and weaning in Mali: cultural context and hard data'. *Social Science & Medicine* 24 (8): 633–644.

Dettwyler K. (1995) 'Beauty and the breast: the cultural context of breastfeeding in the United States'. In: P. Stuart-Macadam and K.A Dettwyler (eds) *Breastfeeding Biocultural Perspectives* (pp. 167–216). New York: Aldine De Gruyer.

DiGirolamo, A.M., Grummer-Strawn, L.M. and Fein, S.B. (2003) 'Do perceived attitudes of physicians and hospital staff affect breastfeeding decisions?' *BIRTH* 30 (2): 94–100.

Dignam, D.M. (1994) 'Understanding intimacy as experienced by breastfeeding women'. *Health Care for Women International* 16: 477–485.

Donnison, J. (1988) *Midwives and Medical Men: A History of the Struggle for the Control of Childbirth.* London: Historical Publications.

Downe, S. and Dykes, F. (in press) 'Counting time in pregnancy and labour', In: C. McCourt (ed.) *Childbirth, Midwifery and Concepts of Time.* London: Berghaun Books.

Doyal, L. and Pennell, I. (1979) *The Political Economy of Health.* London: Pluto Press.

Driscoll, J.W. (1992) 'Breastfeeding success and failure: implications for nurses'. *Clinical Issues in Perinatal and Women's Health* 3 (4): 565–569.

Duckett, L., Henly, S.J. and Garvis, M. (1993) 'Predicting breast-feeding duration during the postpartum hospitalization'. *Western Journal of Nursing Research* 15 (2): 177–198.

Duden, B. (1993) *Disembodying Women. Perspectives on Pregnancy and the Unborn.* London: Harvard University Press.

Dumit, J. and Davis-Floyd, R. (1998) 'Cyborg babies – children of the third millennium'. In: R. Davis-Floyd and J. Dumit (eds) *Cyborg Babies: From Techno-Sex to Techno-Tots* (pp. 1–21). London: Routledge.

Dykes, F. (1995) 'Valuing breastfeeding in midwifery education'. *British Journal of Midwifery* 3 (10): 544–547.

Dykes, F. (1997) 'Return to breastfeeding: a global health priority'. *British Journal of Midwifery* 5 (6): 344–349.

Dykes, F. (2002) 'Western medicine and marketing – construction of an insufficient milk syndrome', *Health Care for Women International* 23 (5): 492–502.

Dykes, F. (2003) *Infant Feeding Initiative: A Report Evaluating the Breastfeeding Practice Projects 1999–2002.* London: Department of Health. At: http://www.dh.gov.uk/assetRoot/04/08/44/59/04084459.pdf (accessed 9 November 2004).

Dykes, F. (2005a) '"Supply" and "Demand": Breastfeeding as Labour'. *Social Science & Medicine* 60 (10): 2283–2293.

Dykes, F. (2005b) 'A critical ethnographic study of encounters between midwives and breastfeeding women on postnatal wards'. *Midwifery* 21: 241–252.

Dykes, F. (2005c) 'Government funded breastfeeding peer support projects: Implications for practice'. *Maternal & Child Nutrition* 1: 21–31.

Dykes, F. and Griffiths, H. (1998) 'Societal influences upon initiation and continuation of breastfeeding'. *British Journal of Midwifery* 6 (2): 76–80.

Dykes, F. and Hall Moran, V. (2003) 'Disadvantaged at birth or by life? An analysis of the relationship between socio-economic factors, in-utero environment and later health'. *Pediatric Research* 53 (6).

Dykes, F. and Hall Moran, V. (2006) 'Transmitted nutritional deprivation: a socio-biological perspective'. In: V. Hall Moran and F. Dykes (eds) *Maternal and Infant Nutrition & Nurture: Controversies and Challenges*. London: Quay Books.

Dykes, F., Hall Moran, V., Burt, S., Edwards, J. and Whitmore, M. (2003) 'Adolescent mothers and breastfeeding – experiences and support needs: an exploratory study'. *Journal of Human Lactation* 19 (4): 391–401.

Dykes, F. and Williams, C. (1999) '"Falling by the wayside": A phenomenological exploration of perceived breast milk inadequacy in lactating women'. *Midwifery* 15: 232–246.

Earle, S. (2000) 'Why some women do not breastfeed: bottle feeding and father's role'. *Midwifery* 16: 323–330.

Ebrahim, G.L. (1991) *Breastfeeding, the Biological Option*. London and Basingstoke: Macmillan.

Edwards, N. (1998) 'Getting to know midwives'. *MIDIRS* 8 (2): 160–163.

Edwards, N. (2000) 'Women planning homebirths: their views on their relationships with midwives'. In: M. Kirkham (ed.) *The Midwife–Mother Relationship* (pp. 55–91). London: Macmillan.

Edwards, N. (2001) 'Women's experiences of planning home births in Scotland – Birthing autonomy'. Unpublished thesis, University of Sheffield.

Edwards, N. (2005) *Birthing Autonomy: Women's Experiences of Planning Home Births*. Oxon: Routledge.

Edwards, R. and Ribbens, J. (1998) 'Living on the edges, public knowledge, private lives, personal experience'. In: J. Ribbens and R. Edwards (eds) *Feminist Dilemmas in Qualitative Research* (pp. 1–23). London: Sage.

Ehrenreich, B. and English, D. (1979) *For Her Own Good, 150 Years of the Experts' Advice to Women*. London: Pluto Press.

Eldredge, J. and Eldredge, S. (2005) *Captivating: Unveiling the Mystery of a Woman's Soul*. California: Nelson Books.

Ely, M., Anzul, M., Friedman, T., Garner, D. and McCormack Steinmetz, A. (1991) *Doing Qualitative Research: Circles Within Circles*. London: Falmer Press.

Engel, G.L. (1977) 'The need for a new medical model: a challenge for biomedicine'. *Science* 196: 129–136.

Engel, G.L. (1980) 'The clinical application of the biopsychosocial model'. *American Journal of Psychiatry* 137 (5): 535–544.

Fairbank, L., O'Meara, S., Renfrew, M.J., Woolridge, M., Sowden, A.J. and Lister-Sharp, D. (2000) 'A systematic review to evaluate the effectiveness of interventions to promote the initiation of breastfeeding'. *Health Technology Assessment* 4 (25).

Fairbank, L., Lister-Sharpe, D., Renfrew, M.J., Wooldridge, M.W., Sowden, A.J.S. and O'Meara, S. (2002) 'Interventions for promoting the initiation of breastfeeding' (Cochrane Review) In: *The Cochrane Library*, Volume 1. Oxford: Update Software.

Fairclough, N. (1992) *Discourse and Social Change*. Cambridge: Polity Press.

Fenwick, J., Barclay, L. and Schmied, V. (1999) 'Activities and interactions in level II nurseries: a report of an ethnographic study'. *Journal of Perinatal and Neonatal Nursing* 13 (1): 53–65.

Fenwick, J., Barclay, L. and Schmied, V. (2000) 'Interactions in neonatal nurseries: women's perceptions of nurses and nursing'. *Journal of Neonatal Nursing*, 6 (6): 197–203.

Fenwick, J., Barclay, L. and Schmied, V. (2001) '"Chatting": an important clinical tool to facilitate mothering in the neonatal nursery'. *Journal of Advanced Nursing* 33 (5): 583–593.

Fildes, V. (1986) *Breasts, Bottles and Babies: A History of Infant Feeding*. Edinburgh: University Press.

Filshie, S., Williams, J., Osborn, M., Senior, O.E., Symonds, E.M. and Backett, E.M. (1981) 'Post-natal care in hospital – time for change'. *International Journal of Nursing Studies*, 18 (2): 89–95.

Fisher, C. (1985) 'How did we go wrong with breast feeding?' *Midwifery* 1: 48–51.

Flagler, S. (1990) 'Relationship between stated feelings and measures of maternal adjustment'. *Journal of Gynaecological and Neonatal Nursing* 19 (5): 411–416.

Fleming, V. (1998a) 'Women and midwives in partnership: a problematic relationship?' *Journal of Advanced Nursing* 27: 8–14.

Fleming, V. (1998b) 'Women-with-midwives-with-women: a model of interdependence'. *Midwifery* 14: 137–143.

Fleming, V. (2000) 'The midwifery partnership in New Zealand: past history or new way forward?' In: M. Kirkham (ed.) *The Midwife-Mother Relationship* (pp. 193–206). London: Macmillan.

Fletcher, D. and Harris, H. (2000) 'The implementation of the HOT program at the Royal Women's Hospital'. *Breastfeeding Review* 8 (1): 19–23.

Foley, P. (1998) 'Reconfiguring knowledge: A discourse analysis of antenatal care'. Unpublished thesis, Bradford University.

Fontana, A. and Frey, J. (1994) 'Interviewing: the art of science'. In: N. Denzin and Y. Lincoln (eds) *Handbook of Qualitative Research* (pp. 361–376). London: Sage.

Ford, G. (1999) *The Contented Baby Book*. London: Vermilion.

Forman, F.J. (1989) 'Feminizing time: an introduction'. In: F.J. Forman and C. Sowton (eds) *Taking Our Time: Feminist Perspectives on Temporality* (pp. 1–10). Oxford: Pergamon press.

Forman, F.J. and Sowton, C. (eds) (1989) *Taking Our Time: Feminist Perspectives on Temporality*. Oxford: Pergamon.

Foster, K., Lader, D. and Cheesbrough, S. (1997) *Infant Feeding 1995*. London: Social Survey Division of the Office for National Statistics.

Foucault, M. (1976) *The Birth of the Clinic: An Archaeology of Medical Perception*. London: Tavistock.

Foucault, M. (1977) *Discipline and Punish: The Birth of the Prison*. Harmondsworth: Penguin.

Foucault, M. (1980) *Power/Knowledge. Selected Interviews and Other Writings by Michel Foucault 1972–1977*. London: The Harvester Press.

Foucault, M. (1981) *The History of Sexuality: An Introduction*. London: Tavistock.

Fox, M. (1989) 'Unreliable allies: subjective and objective time in childbirth'. In: F.J. Forman and C. Sowton (eds) *Taking Our Time: Feminist Perspectives on Temporality* (pp. 123–134). Oxford: Pergamon.

Frank, A.W. (1990) 'Bringing bodies back in: a decade review'. *Theory, Culture and Society* 7: 131–162.

Frank, D., Wirtz, S., Sorenson, J. and Heeren, T. (1987) 'Commercial discharge packs and breastfeeding counselling: effects on infant-feeding practices in a randomized trial'. *Pediatrics* 80 (6): 845–854.

Frankenberg, R. (1980) 'Medical anthropology and development: a theoretical perspective'. *Social Science and Medicine* 14B: 197–207.

Frankenberg, R. (1992a) (ed.) *Time, Health and Medicine*. London: Sage.

Frankenberg, R. (1992b) '"Your time or mine": temporal contradictions of biomedical practice'. In: R. Frankenberg (ed.) *Time, Health and Medicine* (pp. 1–30). London: Sage.

Franklin, S. (1991) 'Fetal fascinations: new dimensions to the medical-scientific construction of fetal personhood'. In: S. Franklin, C. Lury and J. Stacey (eds) *Off-Centre: Feminism and Cultural Studies* (pp. 190–205). London: Harper Collins.

Franklin, S. (1997) *Embodied Progress – A Cultural Account of Assisted Conception*. London: Routledge.

Fraser, D.M. and Cullen, L. (2003) 'Post-natal management and breastfeeding'. *Current Obstetrics and Gynaecology* 13: 127–133.

Freire, P. (1972) *Pedagogy of the Oppressed*. Harmondsworth: Penguin.

Galtry, J. (1997a) 'Suckling and silence in the USA: the costs and benefits of breastfeeding'. *Feminist Economics* 3 (3): 1–24.

Galtry, J. (1997b) 'Sameness and suckling: infant feeding, feminism, and a changing labour market'. *Women's Studies Journal* 13 (1): 65–88.

Galtry, J. (1997c) 'Lactation and the labour market: breastfeeding, labour market changes, and public policy in the United States'. *Health Care for Women International* 18: 467–480.

Galtry, J. (2000) 'Extending the "bright light" feminism, breastfeeding, and the workplace in the United States'. *Gender and Society* 14 (2): 295–317.

Galtry J. (2003) 'The impact on breastfeeding of labour market policy and practice in Ireland, Sweden and the USA'. *Social Science and Medicine* 57: 167–177.

Garcia, J., Redshaw, M., Fitzsimmons, B. and Keene, J. (1998) *First Class Delivery: A National Survey of Women's Views of Maternity Care*. Oxon: Audit Commission.

Garforth, S. and Garcia, J. (1989) 'Breastfeeding policies in practice – "no wonder they get confused"'. *Midwifery* 5: 75–83.

Gaskin, I.M. (1990) *Spiritual Midwifery*. (3rd edn). Summertown: The Book Publishing Co.

George, S. (1994) *A Fate Worse than Debt*. London: Penguin.

Gerrard, A. (2001) 'Breast-feeding in Norway: where did they go right?' *British Journal of Midwifery* 9 (5): 294–300.

Gill, S. (2001) 'The little things: perceptions of breastfeeding support'. *Journal of Gynaecology and Neonatal Nursing* 30 (4): 401–409.

Goer, H. (1995) *Obstetric Myths Versus Research Realities: A Guide to the Medical Literature*. London: Bergin and Garvey.

Gordan, C. (1980) 'Afterword'. In: M. Foucault (1980) *Power/Knowledge. Selected Interviews and Other Writings by Michel Foucault 1972–1977* (pp. 229–259). London: Harvester.

Gough, I. (1979) *The Political Economy of the Welfare State*. London: Macmillan.

Gramsci, A. (1971) *Selections from Prison Notebooks*. London: Lawrence and Wishart.

Grant, J.P. (1995) *The State Of The World's Children*. New York: Oxford University Press for UNICEF.

Gray, A. (1993) 'Health in a world of wealth and poverty'. In: A. Gray (ed.) *World Health And Disease* (pp. 81–97). Buckingham: Open University Press.

Green, J.M., Curtis, P., Price, H. and Renfrew, M. (1998) *Continuing to Care: The Organization of Midwifery Services in the UK: A Structured Review of the Evidence*. Cheshire: Books for Midwives Press.

Greiner, T., Van Esterik, P., Latham, M. (1981) 'The insufficient milk syndrome: an alternative explanation'. *Medical Anthropology* 2: 233–260.

Grossman, L.K., Harter, C. and Kay, A. (1990) 'The effect of postpartum lactation coun-selling on the duration of breastfeeding in low-income women'. *American Journal of Diseases in Childhood* 144: 471–474.

Guba, E.G. and Lincoln, Y.S. (1994) Competing Paradigms in Qualitative Research. In: N. Denzin and Y. Lincoln (eds) *Handbook of Qualitative Research* (pp. 105–117). London: Sage Publications.

Habermas, J. (1972) *Knowledge and Human Interests.* London: Heinnemann.

Halford, S. and Leonard, P. (2003) 'Space and place in the construction and performance of gendered identities'. *Journal of Advanced Nursing* 42 (2): 201–208.

Halldorsdottir, S. (1991) 'Five basic modes of being with another'. In: D.A. Gaut and M.M. Leininger (eds) *Caring: The Compassionate Healer* (pp. 37–49). New York: National League for Nursing.

Halldorsdottir, S. and Karlsdottir, S.I. (1996a) 'Empowerment or discouragement: women's experiences of caring and uncaring encounters during childbirth'. *Health Care for Women International* 17 (4): 135–152.

Halldorsdottir, S. and Karlsdottir, S.I. (1996b) 'Journeying through labour and delivery: perceptions of women who have given birth'. *Midwifery* 12: 48–61.

Hall Moran, V., Dykes, F., Edwards, J., Burt, S. and Whitmore, M. (2005) 'An evaluation of the breastfeeding support skills of midwives and voluntary breastfeeding supporters using the Breastfeeding Support Skills Tool (BeSST)'. *Maternal & Child Nutrition* 1: 241–249.

Hamlyn, B., Brooker, S., Oleinikova, K. and Wands, S. (2002) *Infant Feeding 2000.* London: The Stationery Office.

Hammersley, M. and Atkinson, P. (1995) *Ethnography: Principles in Practice* (2nd edn). London: Routledge.

Haraway, D.J. (1991) *Simians, Cyborgs, and Women: The Reinvention of Nature.* London: Free Association Books.

Hastrup, K. (1995) *A Passage to Anthropology: Between Experience and Theory.* London: Routledge.

Hauck, Y.L. and Irurita, V.F. (2003) 'Incompatible expectations: the dilemma of breastfeed-ing mothers'. *Health Care for Women International* 24: 62–78.

Hauck, Y.L., Langton, D. and Coyle, K. (2002) 'The path of determination: exploring the lived experience of breastfeeding difficulties'. *Breastfeeding Review* 10 (2): 5–12.

Hauck, Y.L. and Reinbold J. (1996) 'Criteria for successful breastfeeding: mother's percep-tions'. *Journal of Australian College of Midwives* 9: 21–27.

Hawkins, A. and Heard, S. (2001) 'An exploration of the factors which may affect the dura-tion of breastfeeding by first time mothers on low incomes – a multiple case study'. *MIDIRS Midwifery Digest* 11 (4): 521–526.

Helman, C. (1992) 'Heart disease and the cultural construction of time'. In: R. Frankenberg (ed.) *Time, Health and Medicine* (pp. 31–55). London: Sage.

Helman, C. (1994) *Culture, Health and Illness* (3rd edn). Oxford: Butterworth-Heinemann.

Helsing, E. (1990) 'Supporting breastfeeding: what governments and health workers can do – European experiences'. *International Journal of Gynaecology and Obstetrics* 31 (Suppl. 1): 69–76.

Henderson, A., Stamp, G. and Pincombe, J. (2001) 'Postpartum positioning and attachment education for increasing breastfeeding: a randomised controlled trial'. *BIRTH* 28: 236–242.

Henderson, L., Kitzinger, J. and Green, J. (2000) 'Representing infant feeding: content analysis of British media portrayals of bottle feeding and breast feeding'. *British Medical Journal* 321: 1196–1198.

Hewat, R. and Ellis, D. (1984) 'Breastfeeding as a maternal-child team effort: women's perceptions'. *Health Care for Women International* 5: 437–452.

Hill, P. and Aldag, J. (1991) 'Potential indicators of insufficient milk supply syndrome'. *Research in Nursing & Health* 14: 11–19.

Hill, P. and Humenick, S. (1989) 'Insufficient milk supply' *IMAGE: Journal of Nursing Scholarship* 21 (3): 145–148.

Hillervik-Lindquist, C. (1991) 'Studies on perceived breast milk insufficiency. A prospective study in a group of Swedish women'. *Acta Pediatrica. Scandinavica* 376: 6–25.

Hillervik-Lindquist, C. (1992) 'Studies on perceived breast milk insufficiency (V): Relation to attitude and practice'. *Journal of Biosocial Science* 24: 413–425.

Hills-Bonczyk, S.G., Tromiczak, K.R., Avery, M.D., Potter, S., Savik, K. and Duckett, L.J. (1994) 'Women's experiences with breastfeeding longer than 12 months'. *BIRTH* 21 (4): 206–212.

Hochschild, A.R. (1979) 'Emotion work, feeling rules and social structure'. *American Journal of Sociology* 85 (3): 551–575.

Hoddinott, P. (1998) 'Why don't some women want to breast feed and how might we change their attitudes?' Unpublished thesis, University of Wales.

Hoddinott, P. and Pill, R. (1999a) 'Qualitative study of decisions about infant feeding among women in east end of London'. *British Medical Journal* 318: 30–34.

Hoddinott, P. and Pill, R. (1999b) 'Nobody actually tells you: a study of infant feeding'. *British Journal of Midwifery* 7 (9): 558–565.

Hoddinott, P. and Pill, R. (2000) 'A qualitative study of women's views about how health professionals communicate about infant feeding'. *Health Expectations* 3: 224–233.

Holloway, I. and Wheeler, S. (1995) 'Ethical issues in qualitative nursing research'. *Nursing Ethics* 2 (3): 223–231.

Hong, T.M., Callister, L.C. and Schwartz, R. (2003) 'First-time mothers' views of breastfeeding support from nurses'. *American Journal of Maternal and Child Nursing* 28 (1): 10–15.

Hoyer, S. and Horvat, L. (2000) 'Successful breast-feeding as a result of a health education programme for mothers'. *Journal of Advanced Nursing* 32 (5): 1158–1167.

Hoyer, S. and Pokorn, D. (2000) 'The influence of various factors on breast-feeding in Slovenia'. *Journal of Advanced Nursing* 27: 1250–1256.

Houston, M., Howie, P. and McNeilly, A. (1983) 'Midwifery Forum 4: Infant feeding'. *Nursing Mirror* 156 (17): supp. i–viii.

Hughes, D., Deery, R. and Lovatt, A. (2002) 'A critical ethnographic approach to facilitating cultural shift in midwifery'. *Midwifery* 18: pp. 43–52.

Humenick, S. and Bugen, L. (1987) 'Parenting roles: expectation versus reality'. *American Journal of Maternal and Child Nursing* 12 (1): 36–39.

Humenick, S.S., Hill, P.D. and Spiegelberg, P.L. (1998) 'Breastfeeding and health professional encouragement'. *Journal of Human Lactation* 14 (4): 305–310.

Humm, M. (1992) *Feminisms: A Reader.* London: Harvester Wheatsheaf.

Hunt, S.C. and Symonds, A. (1995) *The Social Meaning of Midwifery.* Basingstoke: Macmillan.

Hunter, B. (1999) 'Oral history and research part 2: current practice'. *British Journal of Midwifery* 7 (8): 481–484.

Hunter, B. (2001) 'Emotion work in midwifery: a review of current knowledge'. *Journal of Advanced Nursing* 34 (4): 436–444.

Hunter, B. (2002) 'Emotion work in midwifery: an ethnographic study of the emotional work undertaken by a sample of student and qualified midwives in Wales'. Unpublished thesis, University of Wales.

Hunter, B. (2004) 'Conflicting ideologies as a source of emotion work in midwifery'. *Midwifery* 20: 261–272.

Hunter, B. (2005) 'Emotion work and boundary maintenance in hospital-based midwifery'. *Midwifery* 21: 253–266.

Hutchinson, S. (1990) 'Responsible subversion: a study of rule-bending among nurses'. *Scholarly Inquiry for Nursing Practice: An International Journal* 4 (1): 3–17.

Illich, I. (1995) *Limits to Medicine. Medical Nemesis: The Expropriation of Health* (2nd edn). London: Marion Boyars.

Illingworth, R.S. and Stone, D.G.H. (1952) 'Self-demand feeding in a maternity unit'. *The Lancet* 1: 683–687.

Ingram, J., Johnson, D. and Greenwood, R. (2002) 'Breastfeeding in Bristol: teaching good positioning, and support from fathers and families'. *Midwifery* 18: 87–101.

International Baby Food Action Network (IBFAN) (1993) *Protecting Infant Health. A Health Workers Guide to the International Code of Marketing of Breast Milk Substitutes*. Malaysia: International Organisation of Consumers Unions.

Jelliffe, D.B. (1972) 'Commerciogenic Malnutrition'. *Nutrition Reviews* 30 (9): 199–205.

Jelliffe, D.B. and Jelliffe, E.F.P. (1978) *Human Milk in the Modern World*. Oxford: Oxford University Press.

Jenkins, C.L., Orr-Ewing, A.K. and Heywood, P.F. (1984). 'Cultural aspects of early childhood growth and nutrition among the Amele of lowland Papua New Guinea'. *Ecology of Food and Nutrition* 14, 261–275.

Johanson, R., Newburn, M. and MacFarlane, A. (2002) 'Has medicalisation of childbirth gone too far?' *British Medical Journal* 321: 892–895.

Johnson, M. (1997) *Nursing Power and Social Judgement*. Aldershot: Ashgate.

Jolly, M. (1998) 'Introduction: Colonial and postcolonial plots in histories of maternities and modernities'. In: M. Jolly and R. Kalpana (eds) *Maternities and modernities. Colonial and postcolonial experiences in Asia and the Pacific* (pp. 1–25). Cambridge: Cambridge University Press.

Jordan, B. (1997) 'Authoritative knowledge and its construction'. In: R.E. Davis-Floyd and C.F. Sargent (eds) *Childbirth and Authoritative Knowledge* (pp. 55–79). London: University of California Press.

Kahn, R.P. (1989) 'Women and time in childbirth and during lactation'. In: F.J. Forman and C. Sowton (eds) *Taking Our Time: Feminist Perspectives on Temporality* (pp. 20–36) Oxford: Pergamon.

Kapferer, B. (1988) 'Gramsci's body and a critical medical anthropology'. *Medical Anthropology Quarterly* 2 (4): 426–432.

Kaplan, S.H., Greenfield, S., Gandek, B., Rogers, W.H. and Ware, J.E. (1996) 'Characteristics of physicians with participatory decision-making styles'. *Annals of Internal Medicine* 124 (5): 497–504.

Kaufmann, T. (2000) 'Life after birth: reprioritising postnatal care'. *RCM Midwives Journal* 3 (11): 338–339.

Kavanagh, K., Mead, L., Meier, P. and Mangurten, H. (1995) 'Getting enough: mother's concerns about breastfeeding a preterm infant after discharge'. *Journal of Gynaecological and Neonatal Nursing* 24 (1): 23–32.

Kendall, G. and Wickham, G. (1999) *Using Foucault's Methods.* London: Sage.

Kendall-Tackett, K.A. and Sugarman, M. (1995) 'The social consequences of long-term breastfeeding'. *Journal of Human Lactation* 11 (3): 179–183.

Kincheloe, J.L. and McLaren, P.L. (1994) 'Rethinking critical theory and qualitative research'. In: Denzin, N.K. and Lincoln, Y.S. (eds) *Handbook of Qualitative Research* (pp. 138–157). London: Sage.

King, F.T. (1913) *Feeding and Care of the Baby.* London: Macmillan.

Kirkham, M. (1983) 'Labouring in the dark: limitations on the giving of information to enable patients to orientate themselves to the likely events and timescale of labour'. In J. Wilson-Barnett (ed.) *Nursing Research: Ten Studies in Patient Care* (pp. 81–99). Chichester: John Wiley.

Kirkham, M. (1989) 'Midwives and information-giving during labour'. In: S. Robinson and A.M. Thompson (eds) *Midwives, Research and Childbirth (Volume 1)* (pp. 117–138). London: Chapman and Hall.

Kirkham, M. (1993) 'Communication in midwifery'. In: J. Alexander, V. Levy and S. Roch (eds) *Midwifery Practice. A Research-based Approach.* (pp. 1–19). London: Macmillan.

Kirkham, M. (1997a) 'Labouring in the dark: limitations on the giving of information to enable patients to orientate themselves to the likely events and timescale of labour'. In: P. Abbott and R. Sapsford (eds) *Research into Practice: A Reader for Nurses and the Caring Professions* (2nd edn) (pp. 5–18). Buckingham: Open University Press.

Kirkham, M. (1997b) 'Stories and childbirth'. In: M.J. Kirkham and E.R. Perkins (eds) *Reflections on Midwifery.* London: Balliere Tindall.

Kirkham, M. (1999) 'The culture of midwifery in the National Health Service in England'. *Journal of Advanced Nursing* 30 (3): 732–739.

Kirkham, M. (ed.) (2000a) *The Midwife–Mother Relationship.* London: Macmillan.

Kirkham, M. (2000b) 'How can we relate?' In: M. Kirkham (ed.) *The Midwife–Mother Relationship* (pp. 227–249). London: Macmillan.

Kirkham, M. and Stapleton, H. (2000) 'Midwives' support needs as childbirth changes'. *Journal of Advanced Nursing* 32 (2): 465–472.

Kirkham, M. and Stapleton, H. (eds) (2001a) *Informed Choice in Maternity Care: An Evaluation of Evidence Based Leaflets.* University of York, York: NHS Centre for Reviews and Dissemination.

Kirkham, M. and Stapleton, H. (2001b) 'The culture of maternity care'. In: M. Kirkham and H. Stapleton (eds) *Informed Choice in Maternity Care: An Evaluation of Evidence Based Leaflets* (pp. 137–150). University of York: NHS Centre for Reviews and Dissemination.

Kirkham, M. and Stapleton, H. (2001c) 'The ethnographic study'. In: M. Kirkham and H. Stapleton H (eds) *Informed Choice in Maternity Care: An Evaluation of Evidence Based Leaflets* (pp. 13–22). University of York: NHS Centre for Reviews and Dissemination.

Kirkham, M., Stapleton, H., O'Cathain, A. and Curtis, P. (2001) 'Discussion'. In: M. Kirkham and H. Stapleton (eds) *Informed Choice in Maternity Care: An Evaluation of Evidence Based Leaflets* (pp. 151–162). University of York: NHS Centre for Reviews and Dissemination.

Kirkham, M., Stapleton, H., Thomas, G. and Curtis, P. (2002a) 'Checking not listening: how midwives cope'. *British Journal of Midwifery* 10 (7): 447–450.

Kirkham, M., Stapleton, H., Curtis, P. and Thomas, G. (2002b) 'The inverse care law in antenatal midwifery care'. *British Journal of Midwifery* 10 (8): 509–513.

Kirkham, M., Stapleton, H., Curtis, P. and Thomas, G. (2002c) 'Stereotyping as a professional defence mechanism'. *British Journal of Midwifery* 10 (9): 549–552.

Kitzinger, J.V. (1992) 'Counteracting, not reenacting, the violation of women's bodies: the challenge for perinatal caregivers'. *Birth* 19(4): 219–221.

Koch, T. (1994) 'Establishing rigour in qualitative research: the decision trail'. *Journal of Advanced Nursing* 19: 976–986.

Koch, T. and Harrington, A. (1998) 'Reconceptualizing rigour: the case for reflexivity'. *Journal of Advanced Nursing* 28 (4): 882–890.

Kohler Reissman, C. (1992) 'Women and medicalization: a new perspective'. In: G. Kirkup and L. Smith Keller (eds), *Inventing Women. Science, Technology and Gender* (pp. 123–144). Oxford: The Open University Press.

Kramer, M.S., Chalmers, B., Hodnett, E.D., Sevkovskaya, Z., Dzikovich, I., Shapiro, S., Collet J-P., Vanilovich, I., Mexen, I., Ducruet, T., Shishko, G., Zubovich, V., Mknuik, D., Gluchanina, E., Dombrovskiy, V., Kot, T., Bogdanovich, N., Ovchinikova, L. and Helsing, E. (2001) 'Promotion of breastfeeding intervention trial (PROBIT) – A randomized trial in the republic of Belarus'. *Journal of the American Medical Association* 285: 413–420.

Kramer, M.S. and Kakuma, R. (2003) 'Optimal duration of exclusive breastfeeding' (Cochrane Review). In: *The Cochrane Library* (Volume 1). Oxford: Update Software.

Krogstad, U., Hofoss, D. and Hjortdahl, P. (2002) 'Continuity of hospital care: beyond the question of personal contact'. *British Medical Journal* 324: 36–38.

Kuhn, T.S. (1970) *The Structure of Scientific Revolutions.* Chicago: Chicago University Press.

La Leche League (2003a) *A Brief History of La Leche League International.* At: http://www.lalecheleague.org/LLLIhistory.html (accessed 26 September 03).

La Leche League (2003b) *La Leche League's Philosophy.* At: http://www.laleche league.org/philosophy.html (accessed 26 September 03).

La Leche League (2003c) *La Leche League's Purpose.* At: http://www.laleche league.org/purpose.html (accessed 26 September 03).

La Leche League (2003d) About the *La Leche League Peer Counselor Program.* At: http://www.lalecheleague.org/PeerAbout.html (accessed 26 September 03).

Larkin, V. and Butler, M. (2000) 'The implications of rest and sleep following childbirth'. *British Journal of Midwifery* 8 (7): 438–442.

Lavender, T., Moffat, H. and Rixon, S. (2000) 'Do we provide information to women in the best way?' *British Journal of Midwifery* 8 (12): 769–775.

Lavender, T., Walkinshaw, S.A. and Walton, I. (1999) 'A prospective study of women's views of factors contributing to a positive birth experience'. *Midwifery* 15: 40–46.

Lawler, J. (1991) *Behind the Screens: Nursing, Somology and the Problem of the Body.* Edinburgh: Churchill Livingstone.

Leach, J., Dowswell, T., Hewison, J., Baslington, H. and Warrilow, J. (1998) 'Women's perceptions of maternity carers'. *Midwifery* 14: 48–53.

Leap, N. (2000) 'The less we do, the more we give'. In: M. Kirkham (ed.) *The Midwife–Mother Relationship* (pp. 1–18). London: Macmillan.

Leff, E., Gagne, M. and Jefferis, S. (1994) 'Maternal perceptions of successful breastfeeding'. *Journal of Human Lactation* 10 (2): 99–104.

Lewis, J. (1980) *The Politics of Motherhood: Child and Maternal Welfare in England 1990–1939*. London: Croom Helm.

Lewis, J. (1990) 'Mothers and maternity policies in the twentieth century'. In: J. Garcia, R. Kilpatrick and M. Richards (eds) *The Politics of Maternity Care: Services for Childbearing Women in Twentieth-Century Britain*. Oxford: Clarendon.

Levy, V. (1999a) 'Protective steering: a grounded theory study of the processes by which midwives facilitate informed choices during pregnancy'. *Journal of Advanced Nursing* 29 (1): 104–112.

Levy, V. (1999b) 'Maintaining equilibrium: a grounded theory study of the processes involved when women make informed choices during pregnancy'. *Midwifery* 15: 109–119.

Levy, V. (1999c) 'Midwives, informed choice and power: part 1'. *British Journal of Midwifery* 7 (9): 583–586.

Levy, V. (1999d) 'Midwives, informed choice and power: part 2'. *British Journal of Midwifery* 7 (10): 613–616.

Levy, V. (1999e) 'Midwives, informed choice and power: part 3'. *British Journal of Midwifery* 7 (11): 694–699.

Libbus, K., Bush, T.A. and Hockman, N.M. (1997) 'Breastfeeding beliefs of low-income primigravida'. *International Journal of Nursing Studies* 34: 144–150.

Lincoln, S.L. and Guba, E.G. (1985) *Naturalistic Inquiry*. London: Sage.

Lipsky, M. (1980) *Street-Level Bureaucracy: Dilemmas of the Individual in Public Services*. New York: Russell Sage Foundation.

Lipson, J. (1991) 'The use of self in ethnographic research'. In: J. Morse (ed.) *Qualitative Nursing Research: A Contemporary Dialogue* (pp. 73–89). London: Sage.

Llewelyn Davies, M. (1978) *Maternity Letters from Working-Women*. London: Virago.

Lock, L. (1999) 'Making the journey: a feminist analysis of early postnatal discharge'. Unpublished thesis, University of Technology, Sydney.

Lock, L. and Gibb, H. (2003) 'The power of place'. *Midwifery* 19: 132–139.

Locklin, M.P. (1995) 'Telling the world: low-income women and their breastfeeding experiences'. *Journal of Human Lactation* 11: 285–291.

Locklin, M.P. and Naber, S.J. (1993) 'Does breastfeeding empower women? Insights from a select group of educated, low-income, minority women'. *BIRTH* 20 (1): 30–35.

Lomax, H. and Casey, N. (1998) 'Recording social life: reflexivity and video methodology'. *Sociological Research Online* 3 (2): (1–31). At: http://www.socresonline.org.uk/socreonline/3/2/1.html (accessed 21 November 2004).

Lomax, H. and Robinson, K. (1996) 'Asymmetries in interaction: an analysis of midwife–client talk during the postnatal period'. *Proceedings of 24th Triennial Congress of International Confederation of Midwives* (pp. 252–255). Oslo, Norway.

Lugina, H., Johansson, E., Lindmark, G. and Christensson, K. (2002) 'Developing a theoretical framework on postpartum care from Tanzanian midwives' views on their role'. *Midwifery* 18: 12–20.

Lugina, H., Lindmark, G., Johansson, E. and Christensson, K. (2001) 'Tanzanian midwives' views on becoming a good resource person and support person for postpartum women'. *Midwifery* 18: 267–278.

Lupton, D. (1994) *Medicine as Culture: Illness, Disease and the Body in Western Societies*. London: Sage.

Lupton, D. (1995) *The Imperative of Health: Public Health and the Regulated Body*. London: Sage.

Lupton, D. (1996) *Food, the Body and the Self.* London: Sage.

Lynch, B. (2002) 'Care for the caregiver'. *Midwifery* 18: 178–187.

Lyon, M.L. and Barbalet, J.M. (1994) 'Society's body: emotion and the "somatization" of social theory'. In: T. Csordas (ed.) *Embodiment and Experience: The Existential Ground of Culture and Self* (pp. 48–68). Cambridge: Cambridge University Press.

McConville, B. (1994) *Mixed Messages: Our Breasts in our Lives.* London: Penguin.

McCourt, C., Page, L., Hewison, J. and Vail, A. (1998) 'Evaluation of one-to-one midwifery: women's responses to care'. *BIRTH* 25 (2): 73–80.

McCourt, C. and Percival, P. (2000) 'Social support in childbirth'. In: L.A. Page (ed.) *The New Midwifery. Science and Sensitivity in Practice* (pp. 245–268). London: Harcourt.

McCreath, W., Wilcox, S., Laing, V., Crump, D. and Gilles, J. (2001) 'Improving the number of mothers breastfeeding in the postpartum period'. *Primary Care Update* 8 (1): 41–43.

McKeever, P., Stevens, B., Miller, K-L., MacDonell, J.W., Gibbons, S., Guerriere D., Dunn MS, Coyte PC (2002) 'Home versus hospital breastfeeding support for newborns: a randomized controlled trial'. *BIRTH* 29 (4): 258–265.

Mackin, P. and Sinclair, M. (1999) 'Midwives' experience of stress on the labour ward'. *British Journal of Midwifery* 7 (5): 323–326.

Maclean, H.M. (1989) 'Women's experiences of breastfeeding: a much needed perspective'. *Health Promotion* 3 (4): 361–370.

McLeod, D., Pullon, S. and Cookson, T. (2002) 'Factors influencing continuation of breastfeeding in a cohort of women'. *Journal of Human Lactation* 18 (4): 335–343.

McQueen, A. and Mander, R. (2003) 'Tiredness and fatigue in the postnatal period'. *Journal of Advanced Nursing* 42 (5): 463–469.

Maher, V. (1992a) *The Anthropology of Breastfeeding: Natural Law or Social Construct.* Oxford: Berg.

Maher, V. (1992b) 'Breast-feeding in cross-cultural perspective: paradoxes and proposals'. In: V. Maher (ed.) *The Anthropology of Breastfeeding: Natural Law or Social Construct* (pp. 1–36). Oxford: Berg.

Maher, V. (1992c) 'Breast-feeding and maternal depletion: natural law or cultural arrangements?' In: V. Maher (ed.) *The Anthropology of Breastfeeding: Natural Law or Social Construct* (pp. 151–180). Oxford: Berg.

Mahon-Daly, P. and Andrews, G.J. (2002) 'Liminality and breastfeeding: women negotiating space and two bodies'. *Health and Place* 8: 61–76.

Marchand, L. and Morrow, M.H. (1994) 'Infant feeding practices: understanding the decision making process'. *Family Medicine* 26 (5): 319–324.

Marchant, S. (1995) 'What are we doing in the postnatal check?' *British Journal of Midwifery* 3 (1): 34–38.

Margolis, L.H. and Schwartz, J.B. (2000) 'The relationship between the timing of maternal postpartum hospital discharge and breastfeeding'. *Journal of Human Lactation* 16 (2): 121–128.

Marmot, M. and Feeney, A. (1996) 'Work and health: implications for individuals and society'. In: D. Blane, E. Brunner and R. Wilkinson (eds) *Health and Social Organisation: Towards a Health Policy for the 21st Century* (pp. 235–254). London: Routledge.

Marston, P. and Forster, R. (1999) *Reason, Science and Faith.* East Sussex: Monarch.

Martin, E. (1987) *The Woman in the Body – A Cultural Analysis of Reproduction.* Milton Keynes: Open University Press.

Martin, J. (1978) *Infant Feeding 1975: Attitudes and Practices in England and Wales.* Office of Population Censuses and Surveys, London: HMSO.

Martin, J. and Monk, J. (1982) *Infant Feeding 1980*. Office of Population Censuses and Surveys, London: HMSO.

Martin, J. and White, A. (1988) *Infant Feeding 1985*. Office of Population Censuses and Surveys, London: HMSO.

Martines, J.C., Ashworth, A. and Kirkwood, B. (1989) 'Breast-feeding among the urban poor in southern Brazil: reasons for termination in the first 6 months of life'. *Bulletin of the World Health Organization* 67 (2): 151–161.

Marx, K. (1970) *A Contribution to the Critique of Political Economy*. Moscow: Progress.

Mason, J. (1996) *Qualitative Researching*. London: Sage.

Maternity Alliance (2003) *All change on maternity leave?* At: http://www.ivillage.co.uk/print/0,9688,171090,00.html (accessed 14 October 2003).

Maternity Care Working Party (2001) *Modernising Maternity Care*. London: RCM, RCOG, NCT.

Maternity Services Advisory Committee for England and Wales (1985) *Maternity Care in Action, Parts I, II, III*. London: HMSO.

Mauthner, M. (1998) 'Bringing silent voices into a public discourse'. In: J. Ribbens and R. Edwards (eds) *Feminist Dilemmas in Qualitative Research* (pp. 119–146). London: Sage.

Mauthner, M. and Doucet, A. (1998) 'Analysing maternal and domestic discourses'. In: J. Ribbens and R. Edwards (eds) *Feminist Dilemmas in Qualitative Research* (pp. 39–57). London: Sage.

May, K.A. (1991) 'Interview techniques in qualitative research: concerns and challenges'. In: J. Morse (ed.) Qualitative Nursing Research – A Contemporary Dialogue. (pp. 188–201). London: Sage.

Menzies, I.E.P. (1960) 'A case-study in the functioning of social systems as a defence against anxiety'. *Human Relations* 13: 95–121.

Menzies, I.E.P (1970) *The Functioning of Social Systems as a Defence Against Anxiety*. London: The Tavistock Institute of Human Relations.

Merewood, A. and Philipp, B.L. (2003) 'Peer counselors for breastfeeding mothers in the hospital setting: trials, training, tributes, and tribulations'. *Journal of Human Lactation* 19: 72–76.

Merleau-Ponty, M. (1962) *Phenomenology of Perception*. London: Routledge and Kegan Paul.

Meyer, D.E. and de Oliveira, D.L. (2003) 'Breastfeeding policies and the production of motherhood: a historical-cultural approach'. *Nursing Inquiry* 10 (1): 11–18.

Meyer Palmer, M., Crawley, K., Blanco, I.A. (1993) 'Neonatal oral-motor assessment scale: a reliability study'. *Journal of Perinatology* 8 (1): 30–35.

Miles, M.B. and Huberman, A.M. (1994) *Qualitative Data Analysis* (2nd edn). London: Sage.

Millard, A. (1990) 'The place of the clock in pediatric advice: rationales, cultural themes, and impediments to breastfeeding'. *Social Science and Medicine* 31 (2): 211–221.

Miller, T. (1998) 'Shifting layers of professional, lay and personal narratives – longitudinal childbirth research'. In: J. Ribbens and R. Edwards (eds) *Feminist Dilemmas in Qualitative Research* (pp. 58–71). London: Sage.

Morrow, A., Guerrero, L., Shults, J., Calva, J.J., Lutter, C., Bravo, J., Ruiz-Palacios, G., Morrow, R.C. and Butterfoss, F.D. (1999) 'Efficacy of home-based peer counselling to promote exclusive breastfeeding: a randomised controlled trial'. *The Lancet* 353 (9160): 1226–1231.

Morse, J.M. (1991) 'Negotiating commitment and involvement in the nurse–patient relationship'. *Journal of Advanced Nursing* 16: 455–468.

Morse, J.M. (1994) 'Emerging from the data: the cognitive processes of analysis in qualitative inquiry'. In: J. Morse (ed.) *Critical issues in Qualitative Research Methods* (pp. 22–43). London: Sage.

Morse, J.M. and Bottorff, J. (1988) 'The emotional experience of breast expression'. *Journal of Nurse-Midwifery* 33 (4): 165–170.

Morse, J.M., Havens, G.A. and Wilson, S. (1997) 'The comforting interaction: developing a model of nurse–patient relationship'. *Scholarly Inquiry for Nursing Practice: An International Journal* 11 (4): 321–343.

Mozingo, J., Davis, M., Droppleman, P. and Meredith, A. (2000) 'Women's experiences with short term breastfeeding'. *Maternal Child Nursing Journal* 25 (3): 120–126.

Muller, P. (1974) *The Baby Killer: A War on Want Investigation into the Promotion of Powdered Baby Milks in the Third World.* London: War on Want.

Murphy, E. (1999) '"Breast is best": infant feeding decisions and maternal deviance'. *Sociology of Health and Illness* 21 (2): 187–208.

Murphy, E. (2000) 'Risk, responsibility, and rhetoric in infant feeding'. *Journal of Contemporary Ethnography* 29 (3): 291–325.

Murphy, E. (2003) 'Expertise and forms of knowledge in the government of families'. *Sociological Review* 51 (4): 433–462.

Murphy, E., Dingwall, R., Greatbatch, D., Parker, S. and Watson, P. (1998) 'Qualitative research methods in health technology assessment: a review of the literature'. *Health Technology Assessment* 2 (16).

Nadesan, M.H. and Sotorin, P. (1998) 'The romance and science of "breast is best": discursive contradictions and contexts of breastfeeding choices'. *Text and Performance Quarterly* 18: 217–232.

Navarro, V. (1992) 'Has socialism failed? An analysis of health indicators under socialism'. *International Journal of Health Services* 22 (4): 583–601.

Newman, J. (1990) 'Breastfeeding problems associated with the early introduction of bottles and pacifiers'. *Journal of Human Lactation* 6: 59–63.

Nissen, E., Gustavsson, P., Widstrom, A-M., and Uvnas-Moberg, K. (1998) 'Oxytocin, prolactin, milk production and their relationship with personality traits in women after vaginal delivery or Cesarean section'. *Journal of Psychosomatic Obstetrics & Gynecology* 19: 49–58.

O'Campo, P., Faden, R., Gielen, A.C. and Cheng Wang, M. (1992) 'Prenatal factors associated with breastfeeding duration: recommendations for prenatal interventions'. *BIRTH* 19 (4): 195–201.

O'Driscoll, K., Meagher, D. and Boylan, P. (1993) *Active Management of Labour* (3rd edn). London: Mosby.

Oakley, A. (1986) *The Captured Womb, A History of the Medical Care of Pregnant Women.* Oxford: Basil Blackwell.

Oddy, W.H., Holt, P.G., Sly, P.D., Read, A.W., Landau, L.I., Stanley, F.J., Kendall, G.E. and Burton, P.R. (1999) 'Association between breastfeeding and asthma in 6 year old children: findings of a prospective birth cohort study'. *British Medical Journal* 319: 815–819.

Odent, M. (1992) *The Nature of Birth and Breastfeeding.* London: Bergin & Garvey.

Ollard R. (1967) 'Forward'. In: C.M. Cipolla (1967) *Clocks and Culture 1300–1700.* London: Collins.

Page, L.A. (2000) *The New Midwifery. Science and Sensitivity in Practice*. London: Harcourt.

Pain, R., Bailey, C. and Mowl, G. (2001) 'Infant feeding in North East England: contested spaces of reproduction'. *Area* 33 (3): 261–272.

Pairman, S. (2000) 'Women-centred midwifery: partnerships or professional friendships?' In: M. Kirkham (ed.) *The Midwife–Mother Relationship* (pp. 207–226). London: Macmillan.

Paley, J. (2001) 'An archaeology of caring knowledge'. *Journal of Advanced Nursing* 36 (2): 188–198.

Palmer, G. (1993) *The Politics of Breastfeeding*. London: Pandora.

Pelling, M., Harrison, M. and Weindling, P. (1995) 'The Industrial Revolution 1750 to 1848'. In: C. Webster (ed.) *Caring and Health: History and Diversity* (pp. 38–62). Milton Keynes: Open University Press.

Perez-Escamilla R., Pollitt, E., Lonnerdal, B. and Dewey, K.G. (1994) 'Infant feeding policies in maternity wards and their effect on breast-feeding success: an analytical overview'. *American Journal of Public Health* 84 (1): 89–97.

Peters, M. and Lankshear, C. (1994) 'Education and hermeneutics: a Freirean interpretation'. In: P.L. McLaren and C. Lankshear (eds) *Politics of Liberation. Paths from Freire* (pp. 173–192). London: Routledge.

Philipp, B.L., Malone, K.L., Cimo, S., Merewood, A. (2003) 'Sustained breastfeeding rates at a US Baby-Friendly Hospital'. *Pediatrics* 112e: 234–e236.

Philipp, B.L., Merewood, A., Miller, L.W., Chawla, N., Murphy-Smith, M.M., Gomes, J.S., Cimo, S. and Cook, J.T. (2001) 'Baby-Friendly hospital initiative improves breastfeeding initiation rates in a US hospital setting'. *Pediatrics* 108 (3): 677–681.

Philpin, S.M. (2002) 'Rituals and nursing: a critical commentary'. *Journal of Advanced Nursing* 38 (2): 144–151.

Pizzini, F. (1992) 'Women's time, institutional time'. In: R. Frankenberg (ed.) *Time, Health and Medicine* (pp. 68–74). London: Sage.

Porteous, R.M., Kaufman, K. and Rush, J. (2000) 'The effect of individualised professional support on duration of breastfeeding: a randomised controlled trial'. *Journal of Human Lactation* 16 (4): 303–308.

Prasad, B. and Costello, A.M. (1995) 'Impact and sustainability of a "baby friendly" health education intervention at a district hospital in Bihar, India'. *British Medical Journal* 310: 621–623.

Pujol, J. (1999) 'Deconstructing and reconstructing: producing a reading on "human reproductive technologies"'. In: C. Willig (ed.) *Applied Discourse Analysis* (pp. 1–21). Buckingham: Open University Press.

Quandt, S. (1995) 'Sociocultural aspects of the lactation process'. In: P. Stuart-Macadam and K. Dettwyler (eds) *Breastfeeding Biocultural Perspectives* (pp. 127–145). New York: Aldine De Gruyer.

Raisler, J. (2000) 'Against the odds: breastfeeding experiences of low income mothers'. *Journal of Midwifery and Women's Health* 45 (3): 253–263.

Rajan, L. (1993) 'The contribution of professional support, information and consistent correct advice to successful breastfeeding'. *Midwifery* 9: 197–209.

Ray, M. (1994) 'The richness of phenomenology: philosophic, theoretic, and methodologic concerns'. In: J. Morse (ed.) *Critical issues in Qualitative Research Methods* (pp. 116–133). London: Sage.

Rea, F., Venancio, S.I., Martines, J.C. and Savage, F. (1999) 'Counselling on breastfeeding: assessing knowledge and skills'. *Bulletin of the World Health Organisation* 77 (6): 492–498.

Redman, S., Watkins, J., Evans, L. and Lloyd, D. (1995) 'Evaluation of an Australian intervention to encourage breastfeeding in primiparous women'. *Health Promotion International* 10 (2): 101–113.

Renfrew, M.J. (1989) 'Positioning the baby at the breast: more than a visual skill'. *Journal of Human Lactation* 5 (1): 13–15.

Renfrew, M.J., Lang, S. and Wooldridge, M.W. (2003) 'Early versus delayed initiation of breastfeeding' (Cochrane Review). In: *The Cochrane Library* (Volume 1). Oxford: Update Software.

Renfrew, M.J., Woolridge, M.W. and Ross McGill, H. (2000) *Enabling Women to Breastfeed. A review of practices which promote or inhibit breastfeeding – with evidence-based guidance for practice.* Mother and Infant Research Unit, University of Leeds. London: The Stationery Office.

Ribbens, J. (1998) 'Hearing my feeling voice? An autobiographical discussion of motherhood'. In: J. Ribbens and R. Edwards (eds) *Feminist Dilemmas in Qualitative Research* (pp. 24–38). London: Sage.

Rice, P.L. (2000) 'Rooming-in and cultural practices: choice or constraint?' *Journal of Reproductive and Infant Psychology* 18 (1): 24–32.

Rice, P.L., Naksook, C., Watson, L. (1999) 'The experience of postpartum hospital stay and returning home among Thai mothers in Australia'. *Midwifery* 15: 47–57.

Righard, L. (1998) 'Are breastfeeding problems related to incorrect breastfeeding technique and the use of pacifiers and bottles?' *BIRTH* 25 (1): 40–44.

Righard, L. and Alade, M. (1990) 'Effect of delivery room routines on success of first breast-feed'. *The Lancet* 336: 1105–1107.

Righard, L. and Alade, M. (1992) 'Sucking technique and its effect on success of breastfeeding'. *Birth* 19: 185–9.

Rodriguez-Frazier, R. and Frazier, L. (1995) 'Cultural paradoxes relating to sexuality and breastfeeding'. *Journal of Human Lactation* 11 (2): 111–115.

Rogers, C. (1961) *On Becoming a Person.* Boston: Houghton Milton.

Rotch, T.M. (1890) 'The management of human breast-milk in cases of difficult infantile digestion'. *American Pediatric Society* 2: 88–101.

Royal College of Midwives (2000a) *Vision 2000.* London: RCM.

Royal College of Midwives (2000b) *Life after Birth: Reflections on Postnatal Care.* London: RCM.

Royal College of Midwives (2002) *Successful Breastfeeding.* London: RCM and Harcourt.

Saadeh, R. and Akre, J. (1996) 'Ten steps to successful breastfeeding: a summary of the rationale and scientific evidence'. *BIRTH* 23 (3): 154–160.

Sachs, M. (2005) '"Following the Line": An ethnographic study of the influence of routine baby weighing on breastfeeding women in the North West of England'. Unpublished thesis, University of Central Lancashire.

Sandall, J. (1997) 'Midwives' burnout and continuity of care'. *British Journal of Midwifery* 5 (2): 106–111.

Sandelowski, M. (1993) 'Rigor or rigor mortis: the problem of rigor in qualitative research revisited'. *Advances in Nursing Science* 16 (2): 1–8.

Sarafino, E.P. (1994) *Health Psychology: Biopsychosocial Interactions.* New York: John Wiley & Sons.

Savage, J. (2000) 'Ethnography and health care'. *British Medical Journal* 321: 1400–1402.

Schmied, V. (1998) 'Blurring the Boundaries. Breastfeeding as Discursive Construction and Embodied Experience'. Unpublished thesis, University of Technology, Sydney.

Schmied, V. and Barclay, L. (1999) 'Connection and pleasure, disruption and distress: women's experience of breastfeeding'. *Journal of Human Lactation.* 15 (4): 325–334.

Schmied, V., Sheehan, A. and Barclay, L. (2001) 'Contemporary breast-feeding policy and practice: implications for midwives'. *Midwifery* 17: 44–54.

Schwarz, E.W. (1990) 'The engineering of childbirth: a new obstetric programme as reflected in British obstetric textbooks, 1960–1980'. In: J. Garcia, R. Kilpatrick and M. Richards (eds) *The Politics of Maternity Care* (pp. 47–60). Oxford: Oxford University Press.

Schy, D.S., Folker Maglaya, C., Mendelson, S.G., Race, K.E.H. and Ludwig-Beymer, P. (1996) 'The effects of in-hospital lactation education on breastfeeding practice'. *Journal of Human Lactation* 12 (2): 117–121.

Segura-Millan, S., Dewey, K. and Perez-Escamilla, R. (1994) 'Factors associated with perceived insufficient milk in a low-income urban population in Mexico'. *Journal of Nutrition* 124: 202–212.

Shallow, H. (2001a) 'Part 1. Integrating into teams: the midwife's experience'. *British Journal of Midwifery* 9 (1): 53–57.

Shallow, H. (2001b) 'Part 2. Connection and disconnection: experiences of integration'. *British Journal of Midwifery* 9 (2): 53–57.

Shallow, H. (2001c) 'Part 3. Teams and the marginalization of midwifery knowledge'. *British Journal of Midwifery* 9 (3):167–171.

Shallow, H. (2001d) 'Part 4. Competence and confidence: working in a climate of fear'. *British Journal of Midwifery.* 9 (4): 237–244.

Shaw, R. (2003) 'Theorizing breastfeeding: body ethics, maternal generosity and the gift relation'. *Body and Society* 9 (2): 55–73.

Sheehan, A. (1999) 'A comparison of two methods of antenatal breastfeeding education'. *Midwifery* 15: 274–282.

Sheehan, D., Krueger, P., Watt, S., Sword, W. and Bridle, B. (2001) 'The Ontario mother and infant survey: breastfeeding outcomes'. *Journal of Human Lactation* 17 (3): 211–219.

Shelton, K. (1994) 'Empowering women to breastfeed successfully'. *Breastfeeding Review* 2 (10): 455–458.

Sheridan, V. (1999) 'Skin-to-skin contact immediately after birth'. *The Practising Midwife* 2 (9): 23–27.

Shildrick, M. (1997) *Leaky Bodies and Boundaries: Feminism, Postmodernism and (Bio)ethics.* London: Routledge.

Sikorski, J., Renfrew, M.J., Pindoria, S. and Wade, A. (2004) 'Support for breastfeeding mothers' (Cochrane Review). In: *The Cochrane Library* (Volume 1). Oxford: Update Software.

Simmons, V. (2002a) 'Exploring inconsistent breastfeeding advice: 1'. *British Journal of Midwifery* 10 (5): 297–301.

Simmons, V. (2002b) 'Exploring inconsistent breastfeeding advice: 2'. *British Journal of Midwifery* 10 (10): 616–619.

Simonds, W. (2002) 'Watching the clock: keeping time during pregnancy, birth and postpartum experiences'. *Social Science & Medicine* 55: 559–570.

Sinclair, M. and O'Boyle, C. (1999) 'The childbirth self-efficacy inventory: a replication study'. *Journal of Advanced Nursing* 30 (6): 1416–1423.

Singer, M. (1988) 'Culture, critical theory and reproductive illness behaviour in Haiti'. *Medical Anthropology Quarterly* 2 (2): 370–285.

Singer, M. (1990) 'Postmodernism and medical anthropology: words of caution'. *Medical Anthropology* 12: 289–304.

Singh, D. and Newburn, M. (2000) *Women's Experiences of Postnatal Care.* London: National Childbirth Trust.

Slaven, S. and Harvey, D. (1981) 'Unlimited suckling time improves breastfeeding'. *The Lancet,* 1 (8216): 392–393.

Smale, M. (1996) 'Women's breastfeeding: an analysis of women's contacts with a National Childbirth Trust breastfeeding counsellor in England 1979–1989'. Unpublished thesis, University of Bradford.

Smale, M. (2000) 'Women's bodies, women's meanings'. *Barriers to Breastfeeding.* National conference organised by the Royal College of Midwives, the National Childbirth Trust, the Community Practitioners and Health Visitors Association and the Royal College of Nursing. Published proceedings, London: Royal College of Midwives.

Sokol, E. (1997) *The Code Handbook: a Guide to Implementing the International Code of Marketing of Breast-milk Substitutes.* Penang: International Baby Food Action Network.

Spiro, A. (1994) 'Breastfeeding experiences of Gujarati women living in Harrow'. Unpublished MSc Medical Anthropology Dissertation, Brunel University.

Spiro, A. (2006) 'Gujarati women and their infant feeding decisions'. In: V. Hall Moran and F. Dykes (eds) *Maternal and Infant Nutrition and Nurture: Controversies and Challenges* (pp. 232–249). London: Quay Books.

Spradley, J.P. (1980) *Participant Observation.* New York: Holt, Rinehart & Winston.

Stacey, J. (1997) *Teratologies: A Cultural Study of Cancer.* Routledge, London.

Stamp, G.E. and Crowther, C.A. (1994) 'Women's views of their postnatal care by midwives at an Adelaide Women's hospital'. *Midwifery* 10: 148–155.

Standing, K. (1998) 'Writing the voices of the less powerful – research on lone mothers'. In: J. Ribbens and R. Edwards (eds) *Feminist Dilemmas in Qualitative Research* (pp. 186–202). London: Sage.

Stanley, L. and Wise, S. (1993) *Breaking Out Again: Feminist Ontology and Epistemology.* London: Routledge.

Stapleton, H. (2000) 'The MIDIRS informed choice leaflets in clinical practice'. *MIDIRS Midwifery Digest* 10 (3): 388–392.

Stapleton, H. and Thomas, G. (2001) 'Information as communicated and used'. In: M. Kirkham and H. Stapleton (eds) *Informed Choice in Maternity Care: An Evaluation of Evidence Based Leaflets* (pp. 89–102). University of York: NHS Centre for Reviews and Dissemination.

Stapleton, H., Kirkham, M. and Thomas, G. (2002a) 'Qualitative study of evidence based leaflets in maternity care'. *British Medical Journal* 324: 1–6.

Stapleton, H., Kirkham, M., Curtis, P. and Thomas, G. (2002b) 'Framing information in antenatal care'. *British Journal of Midwifery* 10 (4): 197–201.

Stapleton, H., Kirkham, M., Thomas, G. and Curtis, P. (2002c) 'Language use in antenatal consultations'. *British Journal of Midwifery* 10 (5): 273–277.

Stapleton, H., Kirkham, M., Curtis, P. and Thomas, G. (2002d) 'Silence and time in antenatal care'. *British Journal of Midwifery* 10 (6): 394–396.

Stapleton, H., Kirkham, M., Thomas, G. and Curtis, P. (2002e) 'Midwives in the middle: balance and vulnerability'. *British Journal of Midwifery* 10 (10): 607–610.

Starkey, K. (1992) 'Time and the hospital consultant'. In: R. Frankenberg (ed.) *Time, Health and Medicine* (pp. 94–107). London: Sage.

Stearns, C.A. (1999) 'Breastfeeding and the good maternal body'. *Gender and Society* 13 (3): 308–325.

Stein, J., Dykes, F. and Bramwell, R. (2000) 'Breastfeeding: midwives meeting mothers in the middle'. *British Journal of Midwifery* 8 (4): 239–245.

Stevens, T. and McCourt, C. (2002a) 'One-to-one midwifery practice part 3: meaning for midwives'. *British Journal of Midwifery* 10 (2): 111–115.

Stevens, T. and McCourt, C. (2002b) 'One-to-one midwifery practice part 4: sustaining the model'. *British Journal of Midwifery* 10 (3): 174–179.

Strauss, A. and Corbin, J. (1990) *Basics of Qualitative Research. Grounded theory procedures and techniques.* London: Sage.

Street, A.F. (1992) *Inside Nursing: A Critical Ethnography of Clinical Nursing Practice.* Albany: State University of New York Press.

Svedulf, C., Ingegerd, L., Engberg, B., Berthold, H. and Hogland, I. (1998) 'A comparison of the incidence of breastfeeding two and four months after delivery in mothers discharged within 72 hours and after 72 hours post delivery'. *Midwifery* 14: 37–47.

Syme, S.L. (1996) 'To prevent disease: the need for a new approach'. In: D. Blane, E. Brunner and R. Wilkinson (eds) *Health and Social Organisation: Towards a Health Policy for the 21st Century* (pp. 21–31). London: Routledge.

Symonds, A. and Hunt, S. (1996) *The Midwife and Society: Perspectives, Policies and Practice.* London: Macmillan.

Tarkka, M.T. and Paunonen, M. (1996) 'Social support provided by nurses to recent mothers on a maternity ward'. *Journal of Advanced Nursing* 23: 1202–1206.

Tarkka, M.T., Paunonen, M. and Laippala, P. (1998) 'What contributes to breastfeeding success after childbirth in a maternity ward in Finland?' *Birth* 25 (3): 175–181.

Tarlov, A. (1996) 'Social determinants of health: the sociobiological translation'. In: D. Blane, E. Brunner and R. Wilkinson (eds) *Health and Social Organisation: Towards a Health Policy for the 21st Century* (pp. 71–93). London: Routledge.

Tew, M. (1995) *Safer Childbirth? A Critical History of Maternity Care.* London: Chapman and Hall.

Thomas, H. (1992) 'Time and the cervix'. In: R. Frankenberg (ed.) *Time, Health and Medicine* (pp. 56–67). London: Sage.

Thomas, J. (1993) 'Doing critical ethnography'. *Qualitative Research Methods* (Volume 26). London: Sage.

Tong, R.P. (1998) *Feminist Thought: A More Comprehensive Introduction* (2nd edn). Oxford: Westview Press.

Townsend, P., Whitehead, M. and Davidson, N. (eds) (1992) *Inequalities in Health: the Black Report and the Health Divide.* London: Penguin.

Ueda, T., Yokoyama, Y., Irahara, M. and Aono, T. (1994) 'Influence of psychological stress on suckling-induced pulsatile oxytocin release'. *Obstet Gynecol* 84: 259–262.

UNICEF UK Baby Friendly Initiative (2001) *Implementing the Baby Friendly Best Practice Standards.* London: UNICEF UK Baby Friendly Initiative.

Van Esterik, P. (1988) 'The insufficient milk syndrome: biological epidemic or cultural construction?' In: P. Whelehan (ed.) *Women and Health Cross-cultural Perspectives* (pp. 97–108). Bolton: Bergin & Garvey.

Van Esterik, P. (1989a) *Motherpower and Infant Feeding*. London: Zed Books.

Van Esterik, P. (1989b) *Beyond the Breast-Bottle Controversy.* New Brunswick, NJ: Rutgers University Press.

Van Esterik, P. (1994) 'Breastfeeding and feminism'. *International Journal of Gynaecology & Obstetrics* 47: S41–S54.

Van Esterik, P. (1995) 'The politics of breastfeeding: an advocacy perspective'. In: P. Stuart-Macadam and K. Dettwyler (eds) *Breastfeeding Biocultural Perspectives* (pp. 145–166). New York: Aldine De Gruyer.

Van Esterik, P. (1996) 'Expressing ourselves: breast pumps'. *Journal of Human Lactation* 12 (4): 273–274.

Van Manen, M. (1990) *Researching Lived Experience. Human Science for an Action Sensitive Pedagogy.* New York: University of New York Press.

Vandiver, T.A. (1997) 'Relationship of mothers' perceptions and behaviours to the duration of breastfeeding'. *Psychological Reports* 80: 1375–1384.

Varcoe, C., Rodney, P. and McCormick, J. (2003) 'Health care relationships in context: an analysis of three ethnographies'. *Qualitative Health Research* 13 (7): 957–973.

Victora, C., Behague, P., Barros, F., Olinto, M. and Weiderpass, E. (1997) 'Pacifier use and short breastfeeding duration: cause, consequence or coincidence?' *Pediatrics* 99 (3): 445–453.

Vincent, P. (1999) *Feeding our babies. Exploring traditions of breastfeeding and infant nutrition.* Cheshire: Hochland & Hochland.

Vincent, R. (1910) *The Nutrition of the Infant.* London: Bailliere, Tindal & Cox.

Vogel, A.M. and Mitchell, E.A. (1998) 'The establishment and duration of breastfeeding, part 1: hospital influences'. *Breastfeeding Review* 6: 5–9.

Waldenstrom, U., Sundelin, C. and Lindmark, G. (1987) 'Early and late discharge after hospital birth: breastfeeding'. *Acta Paediatrica Scandinavica* 76: 727–732.

Wall, G. (2001) 'Moral constructions of motherhood in breastfeeding discourse'. *Gender and Society* 15 (4): 592–610.

Walsh, D. (2006) 'Subverting the assembly-line: childbirth in a free-standing birth centre'. *Social Science and Medicine* 62: 1330–1340.

Waterworth, S. (2003) 'Time management strategies in nursing practice'. *Journal of Advanced Nursing* 43 (5): 432–440.

Webb, C. (1999) 'Analysing qualitative data: computerized and other approaches'. *Journal of Advanced Nursing* 29 (2): 323–330.

Weitz, R. (2001) 'Women and their hair: seeking power through resistance and accommodation'. *Gender and Society* 15 (5): 667–686.

West, J. and Topping, A. (2000) 'Breast-feeding policies: are they used in practice?' *British Journal of Midwifery* 8 (1): 36–40.

Westphal, M.F., Taddei, J.A.C., Venancio, S.I. and Bogus, C.M. (1995) 'Breast-feeding training for health professionals and resultant institutional changes'. *Bulletin of the World Health Organisation,* 73 (4): 461–468.

Whelan, A. and Lupton, P. (1998) 'Promoting successful breastfeeding among women of low income'. *Midwifery* 14: 94–100.

White, A., Freeth, S. and O'Brien, M. (1992) *Infant Feeding 1990.* Office of Population Censuses and Surveys, London: HMSO.

WHO (1981) *International Code of Marketing of Breast-Milk Substitutes.* Geneva: WHO.

WHO (1990) *Innocenti Declaration on the Protection, Promotion and Support of Breastfeeding.* Florence: WHO.

WHO/UNICEF (1992) *Baby Friendly Hospital Initiative Part II. Hospital Level implementation*. Geneva: WHO/UNICEF.

WHO (1994a) *Infant and Young Child Nutrition*. World Health Assembly WHA 47.5. Geneva: WHO.

WHO (1994b) *An Evaluation of Infant Growth*. WHO working group on infant feeding. Geneva: WHO.

WHO (1998) *Evidence for the Ten Steps to Successful Breastfeeding*. Geneva: WHO.

WHO (2001) WHO Resolution 54.2. At: www.who.int/wha-1998/EB_WHA/PDF/WHA54/ea54r2.pdf (accessed 18 May 2004).

WHO (2003) *Global Strategy for Infant and Young Child Feeding*. Fifty-fifth World Health Assembly. Geneva: WHO.

WHO/UNICEF (1989) *Protecting, Promoting and Supporting Breastfeeding: The Special Role of Maternity Services*. Geneva: WHO & UNICEF.

WHO/UNICEF (1997) *Breastfeeding Management: A Modular Course*. London: UNICEF.

Widstrom, A.M., Ransjo-Arvidson, K., Christensson, K., Mattiesen, A-S., Winberg, J. and Uvnas-Moberg, K. (1987) 'Gastric suction in healthy newborn infants'. *Acta Paediatrica Scandinavica* 76: 566–572.

Wiessinger, D. (1995) 'Breastfeeding as the "default infant feeding"'. *Journal of Human Lactation* 11 (2): 81–82.

Wiessinger, D. (1996) 'Watch your language!' *Journal of Human Lactation* 12 (1): 1–4.

Wilkins, R. (2000) 'Poor relations: the paucity of the professional paradigm'. In: M. Kirkham (ed.) *The Midwife-Mother Relationship* (pp. 28–54). London: Macmillan.

Wilkinson, R. (1996) *Unhealthy Societies. The Afflictions of Inequality*. London: Routledge.

Willig, C. (1999a) 'Introduction: making a difference'. In: C. Willig (ed.) *Applied Discourse Analysis* (pp. 1–21). Buckingham: Open University Press.

Willig, C. (1999b) 'Conclusion: opportunities and limitations of "applied" discourse analysis'. In: C. Willig (ed.) *Applied Discourse Analysis* (pp. 145–159). Buckingham: Open University Press.

Wilson, A., Forsyth, S., Greenie, S.A., Irvine, L. and Hau, C. (1998) 'Relation of infant diet to childhood health: seven year follow up of cohort of children in Dundee infant feeding study'. *British Medical Journal* 316: 21–25.

Winterburn, S. and Fraser, R. (2000) 'Does the duration of postnatal stay influence breast-feeding rates at one month in women giving birth for the first time? A randomized control trial'. *Journal of Advanced Nursing* 32 (5): 1152–1157.

Wolf, J.H. (2000) 'The social and medical construction of lactation pathology'. *Women and Health* 30 (3): 93–109.

Woods, A., Dykes, F. and Bramwell, R. (2002) 'An intervention study using a breastfeeding positioning and attachment tool'. *Clinical Effectiveness in Nursing* 6: 134–142.

Woodward, V. (2000) 'Caring for women: the potential contribution of formal theory to midwifery practice'. *Midwifery* 16: 68–75.

Woolridge, M. (1986a) 'The "anatomy" of infant sucking'. *Midwifery* 2: 164–171.

Woolridge, M. (1986b) 'Aetiology of sore nipples'. *Midwifery* 2: 172–176.

Woolridge, M. (1994) 'The Baby Friendly Hospital Initiative UK'. *Modern Midwife* 4 (5): 29–30.

Woolridge, M. (1995) 'Baby-controlled feeding: biocultural implications'. In: P. Stuart-Macadam and K. Dettwyler (eds) *Breastfeeding Biocultural Perspectives* (pp. 168–217). New York: Aldine De Gruyer.

Wright, A. (1996) 'Changing hospital practices to increase duration of breastfeeding'. *Pediatrics* 97 (5): 669–675.

Wright, S. (1998) 'Politicisation of "culture"'. *Anthropology in Action* 5: 3–10.

Wrigley, E.A. and Hutchinson, S.A. (1990) 'Long-term breastfeeding: the secret bond'. *Journal of Nurse-Midwifery* 35 (1): 35–41.

Yelland, J., Small, R., Lumley, J., Rice, P.L., Cotronei, V. and Warren, R. (1998) 'Support, sensitivity, satisfaction: Filipino, Turkish and Vietnamese women's experiences of post-natal hospital stay'. *Midwifery* 14: 144–154.

Zeitlyn, S. and Rowshan, R. (1997) 'Privileged knowledge and mothers' "perceptions": the case of breast-feeding and insufficient milk in Bangladesh'. *Medical Anthropology Quarterly* 11 (1): 56–68.

# Index